Tib-e-Nabvi
Prophetic Medicine Unveiled

Sirin Seif

ABSTRACT

Prophetic Medicine (*Ṭibb al-nabawī*) is an Islamic genre of religious medical literature that mostly developed in Damascus between the 11th to 14th centuries. It is a type of medical writings that gradually incorporated Greco-Islamic medical theory into *ḥadīth* (i.e. reports from the Prophet) compilations that focus on medicine. While modern scholarship focused on the question of the relationship between this genre and the medical science inherited from the Greeks, this thesis argues that Prophetic Medicine should be put back in its context and understood in its authors own terms. The issue of whether it was an attempt to compete with "Hellenistic" medicine advocated in academic medical literature, or whether it attempted to complement it in religious terms, cannot be resolved merely through the framework of the clash between reason and revelation. Indeed, if the naturalistic tendencies of Greek medicine appealed to the Muslims, the sort of medicine that they encountered when reading the Greek authors was far from atheistic and exclusively rational. The context under Seljūk and early Mamlūk rule of the 11th to the 14th centuries was one that stimulated intellectual activity, as well as a sentiment, for certain scholars, that a return to a more original version of Islam was necessary. It is against such convoluted background that Prophetic Medicine must be understood. The development of this genre can be seen as a four-stages evolution where purely religious compilations of Prophetic reports start to include more and more Greek-based medical theory. The end-product of this evolution is a medical literature that engages directly with religious doctrine, sometimes critically, and merges the two traditions to form a stand-alone genre.

TABLE OF CONTENTS

Man has been truly termed a "microcosm," or little world in himself, and the structure of his body should be studied not only by those who wish to become doctors, but by those who wish to attain to a more intimate knowledge of God, just as close study of the niceties and shades of language in a great poem reveals to us more and more of the genius of its author.

- al-Ghazālī

INTRODUCTION

The study of *Ṭibb al-nabawī* ("Prophetic Medicine") in modern scholarship is not very prolific and discussions of it are often presented at most as paragraphs or chapters in monographies and articles treating of more global topics, such as medicine in Medieval Islam. More often than not, Prophetic Medicine comes up when an author interested in Islamic Medicine mentions marginally this relatively obscure child of Religion and Medicine.

The only extensive study of Prophetic Medicine is the work of Irmeli Perho titled *The Prophet's Medicine: A Creation of the Muslim Traditionalist Scholars*, which was published in 1995.[1] It is the most comprehensive modern title, and it addresses many questions pertaining to the history, historiography, and the content of Prophetic Medicine. However, we intend to present here what I will contend is a short-coming of the Perho's work, namely his interpretation of the motives of the Medieval authors of Prophetic Medicine. Perho reviews the early historiography of Prophetic Medicine and provides an exhaustive assessment of the work done in the twentieth century. However, it appears that the gist of his analysis is too deeply rooted in the early revisionist framework of the study of Islamic Sciences, and thus concentrates too much on the question of what Prophetic Medicine contains of Greek medicine, and what these authors owe to Hippocrates and Galen, rather than trying to understand Prophetic Medicine on its own terms.

The main issue that interests the present study is the discussion of the nature of Prophetic Medicine and this mostly pertains to the motives and the circumstances that propelled its

[1] Irmeli Perho, *The Prophet's Medicine: A Creation of the Muslim Traditionalist Scholars* (Helsinki: Studia Orientalia, 1998).

development during the 13th and 14th centuries. To put it simply, did the authors of this genre attempt to create an alternative to the medical system inherited from the Greeks and standardized by the *Canon* of Ibn Sīnā? Or was it rather a relation of complementarity? To assess this issue, Perho's study is a very good starting point because of its exhaustive focus on the content, but we shall attempt to put Prophetic Medicine back into its context, and to locate the factors that made it possible for this type of medico-religious literature to appear in the way that it did. To be sure, this development finds its root in the wake of the very beginning of Islam, and even earlier in the role of religion in ancient Greek medicine.

A holistic approach to the context that eventually led to the appearance and the development of Prophetic Medicine shall make apparent that challenging Greco-Islamic medicine based on Galen's principles was not the dominant aim of this genre. However, as we shall demonstrate, its evolution also demonstrates that it was part of a more widespread reaffirmation of traditionalism and a longing for a return to a more "authentic" version of Islam. Thus, to the question of whether the authors' desire was to compete with Greek medicine, or to complete it, our answer must fall somewhere in the middle.

The sources that we will use for this thesis are mainly secondary sources. This study will also use primary sources, but will focus on edited translations of this type of works. The main works that will be the object of study are the later works of Prophetic Medicine, such as the *Ṭibb al-nabawī* of Shams al-Dīn al-Dhahabī (d. 1348), translated by Cyril Elgood and published in 1962[2] but misattributed to Jalāl al-Dīn al-Suyūṭī (d. 1505), and that of Ibn Qayyim al-Jawziyya (d.

[2] Cyril Elgood, *Tibb-ul-Nabbi or Medicine of the Prophet: Being a Translation of Two Works of the Same Name. I. -- The Ṭibb-ul-Nabbi of al-Suyúṭi, II. The Ṭibb-ul-Nabbi of Maḥmúd bin Mohamed al-Chaghhayni. Osiris 14 (1962): 33-192.*

1350), translated by Penelope Johnstone and published in 1998.[3] The reason for the focus on these works is the level of complexity that they present relative to earlier works. These are among the most exhaustive treatises, and they represent the result of more than five centuries of evolution of what was known as Prophetic Medicine.

The first chapter of this thesis will present an overview of Greek medicine as it was encountered by the Muslims. Some remarks will be made as to characteristics proper to the Galenic heritage that were significant for the way it was adopted by Muslims and interpreted in treatises of Prophetic Medicine. The particularly complicated relationship with religion that typified medicine in Ancient Greece, their interactions and evolution, were instrumental in the way it later related to Islam and to the Sunna. The discipline of medicine indeed had something of the divine, and could not be thoroughly separated from the religious background on which it was developed. It was neither "secular" nor atheistic, but it presented a type of rationalism that could appeal to the monotheistic faith of the Muslims.

The second chapter is a presentation of the political and intellectual context of the 11th to the 14th centuries, and focuses on the factors that were meaningful in the evolution of Prophetic Medicine, particularly in early Mamlūk Damascus. For indeed, our contention concerning the nature of Prophetic Medicine is highly dependent on its evolution, and on the context which gave rise to the developments that took place in the 13th and 14th centuries. The Mongol invasions bring all manner of intellectuals and religious scholars to the region of Syria and Egypt and produces a cultural effervescence. Also, in search of religious and social legitimization, the military elites took different actions and favored certain policies that resulted in the opening of an intellectual arena

[3] Ibn Qayyim al-Jawziyya, *Medicine of the Prophet*, trans. Penelope Johnstone (Cambridge: Islamic Texts Society, 1998).

for groups that took an interest in the defining of orthodoxy, such as the "traditionalists", who were relatively prolific in the genre of Prophetic Medicine. Furthermore, certain groups that were given more space in this period felt that the ruling elite's ethnic background and practices were not satisfactory according to Islamic doctrine and, for some, this prompted the sentiment that a return to a more "original" version of Islam was necessary.

The third chapter offers a chronological study of the main works of Prophetic Medicine and the evolution of their content from its inception in the thematic separation of *ḥadīths* in the first compilations of reports of the Prophet's sayings and actions to the extensive treatises dedicated to the Prophet's medicine constituting a genre of medical literature in and of itself. We separate the development of Prophetic Medicine into four phases, but it should be noted that these phases are merely an analytical tool, and that some examples do not necessarily fit the separations. The first phase, taking place between the 8th and the 9th centuries, is characterized by the formation of the classical corpus of *ḥadīths* in the form of extensive compilations. In order to grasp the medical content of the Prophetic sayings, we shall present an overview of medical *ḥadīths* of the *Saḥīḥ* of Muḥammad ibn Ismāʿīl al-Bukhārī (d. 870). In the second phase, between the 10th and the 12th centuries, the authors of works of Prophetic Medicine start to organize their works differently, henceforth somehow emulating the contemporary medical books in terms of the arrangement and the order of the subject matters. In the third stage, between the 12th and 13th centuries, the texts seem to mutate from simple *ḥadīth* collections to include explanations of medical theory based on Galenic principles. Finally, the fourth and last stage of the development of Prophetic Medicine represents a culmination of this evolution, focusing all the more on Greek inspired medical theory, merging it to the sayings of the Prophet, and even providing religiously informed criticism to the medical theory accepted by its contemporaries.

Before all of this, however, we must first delve into the heart of the historiographical discussions presented in modern research on Prophetic Medicine. The main problematic that surfaces is that of the purpose of these works as conceived in the minds of their authors. Was it aimed at providing an alternative to Graeco-Islamic medicine which dominated the academic medical literature? Did it attempt to complete it by justifying it in religious terms? Or was it simply a transfer of the authority of medical knowledge from the ancient Greeks to the Prophet? On the other hand, was the aim of this genre to compete with "academic" medicine rather than attempt to complete it? Concerning this latter issue, modern authors that dealt with Prophetic Medicine seem not to have reached a consensus.

In 1976, Christoph Bürgel authored an article titled "Secular and Religious Features of Medieval Arabic Medicine" in *Asian Medical Systems: A Comparative Study*, edited by Charles Leslie. In this article, Bürgel's claims belong to an historiography of science in Islam that categorically set reason in opposition to revelation. We shall make some remarks concerning this type of historiography in chapter two of this thesis.

According to Bürgel, Prophetic Medicine was a manifestation of the objection of Muslim religious scholars to the medicine of the pagan Galen. Prophetic Medicine, he claimed, was one of the "several renowned enemies" of rational thought, including "astrology, alchemy and magic."[4] To Bürgel, Prophetic Medicine could not be separated from the issue of whether "rational remedies" and "secular therapies" was compatible with God's omnipotence, and was aimed to act

---

[4] Christoph Bürgel, "Secular and Religious Features of Medieval Arabic Medicine," in *Asian Medical Systems: A Comparative Study*, ed. Charles Leslie (Berkeley: University of California Press, 1976), 54.

as a "counterpart […] to the suspected Galenic medicine."[5] It was "the Islamic dethronement of Galen […] in favor of Bedouin quackery and superstition sanctified by religion."[6]

The sources mentioned by Bürgel in his article are al-Bukhārī's chapters of his *Saḥīḥ*, "On the Sick" and "On Healing" as well as Cyril Elgood's translation of a book of Prophetic Medicine ascribed to Jalal al-Dīn al-Suyūṭī, that was later proven to be that of Shams al-Dīn al-Dhahabī. Bürgel presents an overview of the genre, but does not examine the texts in detail.

For Manfred Ullmann as well, in *Die Medizin im Islam*, Prophetic Medicine was, by its nature, a set of popular practices, magic and superstitions that emerged in the process of competition with the Graeco-Islamic tradition of medicine.[7] To Ullmann, Prophetic Medicine was developed "to counter Hellenistic Greek medicine which for orthodoxy was suspect as being a science of heathen origin."[8] Since medicine had a foreign and impious origin, it was necessary for religious scholars to challenge it with knowledge based on the Revelation.

Fazlur Rahman was the first to voice a counter-argument to this position in 1987 in *Health and Medicine in the Islamic Tradition: Change and Identity*, in which he offers a more thorough discussion of Prophetic Medicine as well as the possible motives of the authors. In this book, he rejects the opinion of Bürgel and Ullmann that Prophetic Medicine appeared in competition to the established Galenic tradition. He puts forward the claim that works of Prophetic Medicine, starting with Ibn al-Jawzī in the eleventh century, did include the principles of Galen, and often cited Ibn Sīnā, Hippocrates and Galen, and that, for this reason, the "Competition" thesis proposed by earlier modern authors does not hold. As we shall see, this was particularly the case of al-Dhahabī and

---

[5] *Ibid.*, 56.
[6] *Ibid.*, 59-60.
[7] Manfred Ullmann, *Die Medizin im Islam* (Leiden: Brill, 1970), 185-189.
[8] Manfred Ullmann, *Islamic Medicine* (Edinburgh: Edinburgh University Press, 1978), 5.

Ibn Qayyim al-Jawziyya and other later authors of the genre, like Muḥammad ibn Mufliḥ al-Maqdisī (d. 1362), who saw the sayings of the Prophet as providing the general principles while the medicine of the doctors "fills in the details."[9]

Further, Fazlur Rahman adds two other possible motivations for the development of Prophetic Medicine. First, he explains that the authors of Prophetic medicine aimed at giving easy access to preventive and curative measures in an act of piety. Thus, he cites an author of the early 15th century, Ibrāhīm ibn ʿAbd al-Raḥmān al-Azraq, who wrote a book of Prophetic Medicine titled *Tashīl al-manāfiʿ fī al-ṭibb wa-al-ḥikma*:

"When I saw that [today] there are few people who concern themselves with medicine but those who seek help from it are many [...], it appeared to deserve a special devotion since no human being can avoid it. Al-Aḥnaf ibn Qais said, 'No intelligent man can afford to abandon three types of knowledge--the knowledge of that which he can take as his provision for the next life, the knowledge whereby he can establish his worldly life which [in turn] will help him establish his faith, and thirdly, such knowledge of medicine as can help repair his ailments.' This, then, motivated me to collect [compile] certain materials concerning this art."[10]

What this shows, according to Rahman, is that there was a pious concern in the aim to popularize the practice of medicine. This pious concern was not merely the dissemination of the Prophet's words and practice, but rather a pious concern for the inevitability of illness and the well-being of his fellow Muslims. Rahman however ends up somewhat conceding to Bürgel,

---

9 Fazlur Rahman, *Health and Medicine in the Islamic Tradition: Change and Identity* (New York: Crossroads, 1989), 43.
10 *Ibid.*, 42

stating that the opposition to "the pagan Galen" might have been a late motive of the development of Prophetic medicine.[11]

The second possible motivation that Rahman ascribes to Prophetic Medicine is that of a spiritualization or an "Islamization" of medical practices that were not properly Islamic or Arab. Some practices came from pre-Islamic Bedouin medicine, others from Greek, Iranian and Indian medicine.

In his review of Fazlur Rahman's book in 1988[12] as well as in his own *Majnūn: The Madman in the Medieval Islamic World* of 1992[13], Michael Dols positioned himself differently from Rahman vis-à-vis Bürgel and Ullmann's theory of the antithetic challenge of Galenic medicine by Prophetic Medicine. Dols objected that this medico-religious literature made its appearance and evolved as it did because it intended to transfer the authority of medical knowledge from Galen to the Prophet without denying the benefits of Galenic medicine. To Michael Dols, this appeared as an Islamic domestication of the scientific medical tradition.[14] He rejected Rahman's claim that the Prophet's medicine could have been a reaction *against* Galenic medicine, but proposed that it was a response to it in the form of an appropriation.

On this debate, Irmeli Perho seems to have the most comprehensive grasp of the different opinions and clearly tips the scale in favor of the opinion of Michael Dols. To the answer of the latter concerning the thesis that Prophetic medicine opposed the Galenic principles of Graeco-Islamic medicine, Perho adds that already early into the existence of the genre, it had adopted the

---

[11] Ibid.
[12] Michael Dols, "Review of *Health and Medicine in the Islamic Tradition: Change and Identity* by Fazlur Rahman," *Middle East Journal* 42, no. 2 (1988): 323-324.
[13] Michael Dols, *Majnūn: The Madman in Medieval Islamic Society* (Oxford: Clarendon Press, 1992).
[14] *Ibid.*, 248.

same organization of subject matters as the contemporary medical books of the doctors. Constant references to Galen, Hippocrates and Ibn Sīnā in the works of al-Dhahabī and later authors like Ibn Qayyīm al-Jawziyya, Ibn Mufliḥ, al-Suyūṭī, etc., show the importance and value of these authors and their ideas, however "un-Islamic" they may have been considered. If a new form of medicine was advocated, it was not to the detriment of the established scientific knowledge.

It is precisely here that we should strive to position our study. It is clear that earlier scholarship did not quite hit the mark in its assessment of the nature of Prophetic Medicine, and Perho's analysis is now almost 20 years old. Meanwhile, the evolution of the discipline of the History of Islamic Science has gone beyond the framework established by pioneering figures of revisionist historiography like Dimitri Gutas, Roshdi Rashed and George Saliba. In the 80s and 90s, these authors challenged the old historiography anchored in the post-Enlightenment idea that reason and science categorically opposed Revelation. However, more recent historians, like historian of Islamic medicine Nahyan Fancy, have critiqued revisionist historiography for its lack of content concerning medicine, and for its focus on the Greek heritage of Islamic science.[15] And indeed, Perho's study seems guilty of the latter: the questions that it strives to answer are along the lines of "How much of Hippocrates', Galen's and Ibn Sīnā's legacies can we identify in works of Prophetic Medicine?" Where the present thesis shall differ from Perho's work is in its focus on contextualisation. In order to grasp and define the nature of the genre of Prophetic Medicine, we must consider its history as a whole.

[15] Nahyan A.G. Fancy, "Pulmonary Transit and Bodily Resurrection: The Interaction of Medicine, Philosophy and Religion in the Works of Ibn al-Nafīs (d. 1288)," (Phd diss., University of Notre Dame, 2006), 17-30.

Chapter 1: From the Greeks to the Authors of Prophetic Medicine

At its beginnings, the genre of literature that carried the name "Prophetic Medicine" took the form of a collection of sayings of the Prophet and of his Companions. The sayings that pertained to medicine could be found in collections of varying nature and form, which we will discuss further below. For now, it is worthwhile to explain that these collections evolved and contained over time a growing amount of Greek medical theory. What came to be known as Prophetic Medicine thus eventually culminated in something that combined the traditions of Islam and the science of the Greeks. By the turn of the 14th century, we see the appearance of treatises of Prophetic Medicine that owe much to the dominant Graeco-Islamic medicine, and thereby to Galen in terms of medical theory, to Dioscorides in terms of pharmacology, Aristotle in terms of philosophy, etc. It thus appears as a prerequisite for us to examine certain aspects of the history of medicine that lead to our period of interest, and that pertain to the Greek medical tradition that was inherited by Muslims.

We will thus need to present the main characteristics of Greek medicine and its connection to the divine, because Prophetic Medicine was essentially a *harmonization* of Galenic-Aristotelian medicine, as distilled in Ibn Sīnā, with the input, or the adjustments, as we will see in chapter 3, of Prophetic *ḥadīth.* We shall discuss Greek medicine's relation to religion for different reasons: (1) the mythological origins of Hippocratic medicine could be interpreted as a form of revelation and therefore rendered relatively more compatible with Islam; (2) Galenic medicine was not "secular" or atheistic, nor was it purely materialistic; (3) at the same time, the naturalistic and “rational” aspect of Greek medicine appealed to Muslims as a way of glorifying God through his creation; (4) Greek medicine had already passed through the hands of Christian students and Syriac translators before being turned into Arabic, and to an extent were "depaganized"; and (5) Muslims had a particularly high regard for the *Oath* and used it in unprecedented ways.

The scientific context of the production of these treatises was marked by the domination of the Islamic adoption and adaptation of Greek medicine inherited from Galen through the intermediaries of the translators of the 8th and 9th centuries. We shall begin this chapter with a brief observation of the interactions between religion and healing in Ancient Greece, for indeed, Muslims did not come into contact with a medical tradition devoid of the influence of religion. The way medicine and religion interacted in Antiquity had repercussions on the conceptualisation of medicine in the works of Muslim physicians, as well as the attitudes of Muslims toward Greek medicine. From the revealed art of the healing god Asclepius and his descendants, the step was not a great one, for Muslim scholars, to claim medicine as the gift of God: one was a legacy of a mythic hero turned god, and the other was the sacred word of God; both were thus seen as revealed knowledge. Then, we will look at the development of rational, naturalistic medicine and its ties to philosophy. We will also present an overview of the conditions of transmission of Greek medical knowledge, the growing influence of Galen during the developments of medicine in an Islamic context starting with the translation movement around the time of the Abbasid caliphate, and the basic principles of Galenic medicine as understood and digested by Ibn Sīnā, as well as Greek ethics of medicine and their impact on the Islamic context. Our goal in this section will be to present the major characteristics of the intellectual legacy of Greek medicine that impinged on Muslim authors of medicine and, by extension, on authors of Prophetic Medicine.

Before we begin it must be acknowledged that the character of medical literature that is presented in this chapter cannot be taken to be completely concordant with medical practice. In late Antiquity, as well as in the Islamic context, the literature that is available to us on medicine that could be called "academic" did not necessarily reflect the actual practice of Galenic medicine.

Religion and Healing in Ancient Greece

When Muslims started to seek out Greek medical knowledge, Galen's (d. ca. 216 CE) medicine was not the only thing that they inherited. The significance of the Greeks', and Galen's, influence was not merely their aetiology based on a quadrumvirate of elements. However, one must grasp an essential factor when putting the confluence of Islam and medicine under the magnifying glass: along with Galen's medical knowledge came a whole *world* of methods, ideas, and ideals, that pertained as much to reason as it did to belief. In this essay, I shall attempt to present a picture of the convoluted world that the Muslims of the late 8th to 9th centuries tapped into during the translation movement.

Ibn al-Nadīm (d. 995), Muslim bibliographer of the 10th century and author of the *Kitāb al-fihrist*, tells us that there were 5560 years between Asclepius and Galen, during which there were eight great "leaders" of medicine, including the famed Hippocrates of Cos (d. 370 BCE).[16] It would not do to attempt to understand Galen without understanding medicine before him, given that his Islamic readers saw him as the heir to a long tradition. Medicine, at the time of Hippocrates, was already a quite intricate reality. Unfortunately, written sources from the pre-Hippocratic

[16] Muḥammad ibn Ishāq Ibn al-Nadīm, *The Fihrist of al-Nadīm; a Tenth-Century Survey of Muslim Culture*, trans. Bayard Dodge (New York: Columbia University Press, 1970), 674-675.

context are relatively scarce and the accounts that we do retain are often incomplete.[17] Some of the gaps are filled by archeological data as well as epigraphic and papyrological remains, but as with much of antique Greek history, we are left to rely on the poems of Homer to give us a sense of medical ideas and practices dating from before any strictly medical literature.[18] In these texts, myth and history converge to bring us an account of an Asclepius, son of Apollo, who was given his knowledge of healing from Chiron the Centaur. Asclepius the hero came to ascend as the Greeks' god of healing in the stead of his father. Homer's narrative of the Trojan wars reports the sons of Asclepius, Machaon and Podalirius to be valued surgeons and medics, *iatros*.[19] While many diseases, especially the ones that affected the masses[20], were viewed as originating from gods as punishments, Machaon, Podalirius and the *iatros* of Greek Antiquity were craftsmen in the likes of armorers, seers, bards, etc. As Vivian Nutton states: "The doctor is [among the] 'servants of mankind at large', whose country 'knows no bounds', and who moves from place to place as and when their services are needed"[21], summoned by rulers to treat them and their relatives, providing treatment to the injured and the sick often without recourse to the gods.[22]

This introduces an aspect of the healing of Asclepius that I would like to emphasize here: the way in which Asclepius performed his healing in the cult centers was remarkably naturalistic. Of course, if there was something miraculous in his treatment, it was its quickness. The recourse to Asclepius by the sick started with the method of incubation, where the patient travelled to a

[17] Vivian Nutton, *Ancient Medicine* (London & New York: Routledge, 2004), 7.
[18] *Ibid.*, 37.
[19] *Ibid.*, 38.
[20] Nutton insists on emphasizing the relativity of this term and explains that what we might perceive as widespread outbreaks of epidemics were actually quite limited in their impacts. While they did affect a great number of people, mass diseases and epidemics in Ancient Greece tended to be more localized than might appear, for the limits of the Mediterranean world were quite impermeable. *Ibid.*, 19-36.
[21] *Ibid.*, 40.
[22] Ibid.

temple dedicated to the god, made the ritual preparations, and slept overnight in the temple. During the night, the patient might dream of being visited by Asclepius, often represented as a snake. Asclepius would either administer a drug, or perform the salutary surgery, or deliver to the patient cryptic messages of recommendations to be interpreted by the priests of the temple upon the waking of the patient. Thus, what is to be stressed here is that Asclepius did not simply magically heal the patient; he most often healed him through naturalistic, somehow "physical", means. While many of the recorded procedures were selected for the impression they would make because of their deviation from expectations, many actually represented convergence with contemporary traditional medicine.[23]

Of course, it would be wrong to describe Asclepius as the only healing god. Vivian Nutton warns us about the danger of exaggerating the dominance of the cult of Asclepius, for indeed, its advent took place relatively late in the scope of Greek history and the temples were generally quite far from the main religious centers.[24] Indeed, in his *Roman Questions*, Plutarch (d. 120 CE) notices the isolation of the temples of Asclepius and proposes that the seperation may have been an attempt to isolate the sick from the rest of the town.[25]

Other gods continued to provide healing to their followers even after the advent of the cult of Asclepius. The cult of Apollo Iatros (the Healer) remained significant in the regions of the Black Sea, and in 433 BCE, merely 13 years before Asclepius first appeared in Athens[26], a temple was erected in Rome for Apollo the Healer. Other gods continued to be revered for their power of

---

[23] Information about these were made available to us through inscriptions that were left by recipients of successful treatments. Indeed, it was customary to repay the god for his help by providing inscriptions to be etched in the very stone of the temple, inscriptions that would detail the treatment and the result. *Ibid.*, 109.
[24] *Ibid.*, 107.
[25] Plutarch, *The Roman Questions of Plutarch: A New Translation with Introductory Essays & a Running Commentary*, trans. H. J. Rose (Oxford: Clarendon Press, 1924), 94: 708.
[26] The first temple of Asclepius in Athens was erected in 420 BCE Nutton, *Ancient Medicine*, 105.

healing such as Zeus, Hercules, and Artemis.[27] In some cases, such as that of Amphiaraus the Hero Healer in Boeotia, the pre-existence of a cult of a healing god hindered the propagation of the cult of Asclepius. This suggests that the latter never came to possess a monopoly over medicine.[28] However, toward the end of the fifth century BCE, with the rise in popularity of his cult and the proliferation of temples dedicated to him, he did become the only god that *specialized* in medicine. The quick accumulation of riches in his temples attests to the increase in supplications to Asclepius and may be linked to many factors: the memory of the plague of Athens of 430 BCE; the influence on other cities of the adoption of the cult in Athens; and the effulgence of the Asclepeion of Epidaurus, the most celebrated healing temple of the Classical world.[29] It is from this context, alongside the development of the cult of Asclepius, that Hippocratic medicine would emerge, and indeed, the mythology of medicine is significant because Hippocrates claimed that he was himself an Asclepiad, i.e. a descendent of Asclepius.

Now for the Muslims, and quite similarly for the Greeks, who saw medicine as the worldly legacy of a hero-turned-god, medicine had originally come from God himself as a revelation. As is shown by the genesis of medicine presented by Ibn al-Nadīm, the myth of the revelation of medicine to Asclepius and his lineage was recognized by Arab physicians as an answer to the question of the theoretical foundations of their art. For Ibn Riḍwān (d. 1061), "medicine had at first been the exclusive possession of the family of Hippocrates," and this view, Strohmaier suggests, was "related to the idea medicine had roots in a sort of revelation."[30] Consequently, this

[27] A Delphic oracle ordered Athenians to sacrifice to Zeus, Hercules and Apollo the Protector in 348 BCE; at Brauron, Artemis was the recipient of the healing vows of young women. *Ibid.*, 107.
[28] *Ibid.*, 107-108.
[29] *Ibid.*, 108-109
[30] Gotthard Strohmaier, "Reception and Tradition: Medicine in the Byzantine and Arab World," in *Western Medical Thought from Antiquity to the Middle Ages*, ed. Mirko D. Grmek et al. (Cambridge: Harvard University Press, 1998), 155-156.

origin of medicine in revelation must have helped defend the art against the attacks of Muslims who were hostile to medicine, and paved the way for the genre of Prophetic Medicine to merge Islamic revelation and Greek medicine. For God was the creator of disease and cure, but "he also revealed (*alhama*) the knowledge of medicaments and guided the way to medical treatment that leads to the cure he has predetermined."[31]

For a Muslim physician like ʿAlī ibn Riḍwān, it was understood that the monopoly over the art of medicine that was claimed by the family of Hippocrates was then disseminated to the general population and thereby deteriorated between the 3rd century BCE and the 2nd century CE. At the hands of Galen, however, the art is said to have been purified and unified.[32] One of the most impactful characteristics of Greek medicine was its rationalism, which we shall discuss in the following section.

Almost simultaneously with the development of the style of religious healing previously discussed, Greece witnessed a revolutionary change that brings medicine closer to the context of its adoption by Arabs. Through this evolution, medicine will come forth as a *techne*, an art. Prior to this, medicine was the privilege of the few, a legacy handed down from father to son, limited to a certain family that claimed ascendance from the sons of Asclepius, the Asclepiads. Medicine, contrary to being an art, was a birthright. To illustrate this development, Jacques Jouanna stresses the significance of the *Oath* of Hippocrates. The importance of this text is undebatable, but it is particularly vital in that it shows the revolutionary opening of the horizons of the art of medicine

[31] Ibn Jumayʿ, *Treatise to Ṣalāḥ ad-Dīn on the Revival of the Art of Medicine*, trans. Hartmut Fähndrich (Wiesbaden: Steiner, 1983), section 14.
[32] Strohmaier, 155.

from the close circle of the Asclepiads, to any and all who would commit to the sacredness of the art as a disciple.[33] Let us unpack this claim. Jouanna is referring here to the first part of the *Oath*:

> "I swear by Apollo the Physician and by Asclepius and by Health [the god Hygieia] and Panacea and by all the gods as well as goddesses, making them judges [witnesses], to bring the following oath and written covenant to fulfillment, in accordance with my power and my judgement;
>
> To regard him who as taught me this techné [art and science] as equal to my parents, and to share, in partnership, my livelihood with him and to give him a share when he is in need of necessities, and to judge the offspring [coming] from him equal to [my] male siblings, and to teach them this techné, should they desire to learn it, without fee and written covenant,
>
> And to give a share both of rules and of lectures, and of all the rest of learning, to my sons and the [sons] of him who has taught me and to the pupils who have both made a written contract and sworn by a medical convention but by no other."[34]

This part of the document is an agreement of community, a contract of association. This is significant because prior to the time of the emergence of the Hippocratic corpus, medicine was said to be the affair of the Asclepiads, descendants of Asclepius who passed on their art from father to son. What this passage represents is the widening, in the 4th century BCE, of the keepers of the art of medicine.

---

[33] Jacques Jouanna, "The Birth of the Western Medical Art," in *Western Medical Thought from Antiquity to the Middle Ages*, ed. Mirko D. Grmek et al. (Cambridge: Harvard University Press, 1998), 28-29.
[34] Steven H. Miles, *The Hippocratic Oath and the Ethics of Medicine* (Oxford: Oxford University Press, 2005), xiii.

Far from being the work of one man, the Hippocratic corpus is the work of many. However, it came to be recognized as *Hippocratic* because its texts and their context converged toward a shared attitude of physicians derived from the teachings of Hippocrates.[35] What Hippocraticism represented was an approach concerning the sick and concerning disease itself based on a humanization and rationalization of causality and clinical observation. The 5th century, according to Jouanna, marked the birth of "humanism" in the broad sense of the term, *i.e.* "man's thought concerning himself and his condition."[36] Indeed, the growing popularity of the cult of Asclepius coincided with an "unprecedented effort in thinking about man in the context of rational factors"[37] and medical thought displayed this evolution by taking the causes of disease away from gods, rejecting or ignoring their intervention, and searching for them in the environment of man.

However, this is not to say that the Greeks suddenly casted out religion in favor of reason. This idea of such a "Greek Miracle" has long since been revised. One of the earliest examples of how religion kept a significant importance in Hippocratic medicine appeared with the Hippocratic treatise *De morbo sacro*. Before Hippocrates, epilepsy, along with the mysterious, sudden, and shocking crisis that it provokes, was explained by the physicians as the result of the direct intervention of the gods. The author attacks his contemporaries for their explanation of the "sacred disease" and suggests that the causes can instead be found in nature, which itself is divine. Changes in the direction and temperature of the winds are responsible for this sickness, and must be counteracted with opposite means.[38] Thus, R.J. Hankinson, in "Magic, Religion and Science: Divine and Human in the Hippocratic Corpus," summed up the essence of the Hippocratic position

---

[35] *Ibid.*, 31-32.
[36] *Ibid.*, 41.
[37] *Ibid.*, 44.
[38] *Ibid.*, 35-40.

concerning the "sacred disease" and the place of the divine in medicine in saying that it is not more divine or sacred than any other disease.[39] *De morbo sacro* depicts an unflattering picture of charlatans who claim to have power over demons and gods by means of chants and charms. Avoiding charges of atheism, the author accuses his contemporaries of impiety when they claim agency over the powers of the gods.[40]

It is not only that nature is divine, but that divinity is also *localized* in nature. The author of *De morbo sacro* did not refute the divinity of the causes of epilepsy, but rejected the possibility that chants and charms could bend nature – and the divine – to the will of mortals. Thus, it is important to acknowledge that Greek medicine, while it takes a turn toward naturalistic aetiology and therapy, continued to be tied to its divine origins. Indeed, as we shall discuss further, Greek medical authors and physicians continued to leave room for the divine and the supernatural: Galen himself recognized the divine foundation of his art, and his commentary on the Hippocratic *Oath* showed as much. We shall also discuss further how Galen's theology remarkably placed divinity in the physical world. And of course, if even the mysterious "sacred disease" could be explained through a physical aetiology, this was a physical world that *contained* the divine: Greek gods were not perceived as transcending the physical world, rather they existed in it, and their agency was in some ways dependant on nature. The author of *De morbo sacro* did not attack the possibility of divine healing, but merely asserted that dietary means were also necessary to ward off disease.[41] "It is one thing," explained Hankinson, "to object to the practices of (at least some of) the diviners, quite another to suppose that medicine should simply eschew all mention of the divine."[42]

---

[39] R. J. Hankinson, "Magic, Religion and Science: Divine and Human in the Hippocratic Corpus," *Apeiron* 31 (2011): 4.
[40] Nutton, *Ancient Medicine*, 113.
[41] *Ibid.*, 113-114.
[42] Hankinson, "Magic, Religion and Science," 4.

Of course, we could not assume that practice followed theory so closely. What this shows is that Greek science, at least in what pertains to medicine, was a pluralistic reality rather than a univocal statement. It was not purely religious or magic, nor was it purely rationalistic and natural. On the one hand, some part of Greek medicine came to be closely associated with natural philosophy, i.e. it suggested an aetiology based on a set of basic principles that pretended to explain all nature. From the earliest philosophers who thought that the world emerged from a single principle, be it numbers for the Pythagoreans, air for Diogenes of Apollonia (fl. 425 BCE), etc., to Empedocles of Agrigentum (d. 430 BCE), who thought that the basic component of the material world were the four elements, to Democritus of Abdera (d. ca. 370 BCE), a great deal of authors of philosophy were also practitioners of medicine or writers of medical theory.[43]

On the other hand, certain authors of medical literature rejected the idea of hypothetical investigation and of overarching principles, for medicine should not be concerned with "the obscure matters in the sky and under the earth but with the afflictions from which people suffer in disease."[44] What is important for us here, is that it is this complex world of interactions between medicine and the divine that could be translated in what came to be known as *al-Ṭibb al-nabawī*. It is in this context, and with these attitudes in mind, that we should think of the Hippocratic corpus[45] and its meaning in the global scope of the history of medicine. Around the 9th century, when the scholars of the Abbasid court started to be interested in Greek sciences, Christian Syriac

[43] Miles, *The Hippocratic Oath*, 46-51.
[44] Hippocrates, *Hippocrates On Ancient Medicine: Translated with Introduction and Commentary*, trans. Mark J. Schiefsky (Leiden: Brill, 2005), 114.
[45] Divided between their geographical origin, the content of the Hippocratic corpus is the following. Among those that originated from Cos, we find a series of treatises on surgery (*De articulis* and *De fracturis*), *Epidemiae*, *De natura hominis*, *De aere, aquis, locis*, *De morbo sacro*, *Prognosticon*, *De diaeta acutorum*, *Aphorismi* and *Praenotiones Coacae*. In the Cnidian school, we have the *Cnidian Maxim* and other nosological treatises such as *De Morbis II* and *III*, etc. Finally, among other texts that were neither from Cos or Cnidus, we find *De carnibus (Regimen)* and *De diaeta*. Jouanna, "The Birth of Western Medical Art", 34-37.

translators such as Ḥunayn ibn Iṣḥāq (d. 873) and his pupils reached out to make the medicine of Hippocrates, complemented by Aristotle and Galen, available to Muslims.

Islamic Reception of Greek medicine: The Historiographical Issue

We have seen how a certain trend of Greek medicine came to embrace causality and define itself by setting the human body, along with the event of disease, firmly in its natural environment, all of this while not thoroughly removing the gods from medicine. With this trend medical theory becomes based on natural causes, and the gods are relatively put aside; however, divinity remains. When early Muslims came into contact with Galenic medicine and Greek sciences in general, certain theologians opposed it on the ground that its insistence on causality could not be reconciled with God's omnipotence. Indeed, if God sends disease to man, what rights and what powers did doctors have to attempt to influence the course of illness?[46] We shall discuss the opinions of certain scholars concerning reliance on God in medicine in the third chapter of this work.

Dimitri Gutas' Greek Thought, Arabic Culture: The Graeco-Arabic Translation Movement in Baghdad and Early 'Abbāsid Society (2nd-4th/8th-10th centuries) (1998) has revealed what he describes as the myth of Islamic opposition to the Greek sciences. This "myth" among modern historians was popularized by the 1916 study of Ignaz Goldziher, "The Attitude of the Old Islamic Orthodoxy toward the Ancient Sciences", published first in German, and translated into English in 1981. According to Gutas, the problem with Goldziher's study was its failure to identify the

[46] Fancy, "Pulmonary Transit and Bodily Resurrection," 14-16.

"orthodoxy"[47] that he pointed at in his title, which gave rise to the overgeneralized misconception that the Muslim theologians who rejected the Greek Sciences constituted an "orthodox" majority.[48] Goldziher's "orthodoxy" was defined backwards through the rejection of Greek Sciences: instead of looking at the many meanings of orthodoxy in Islam and determining which groups accepted it and which groups didn't, Goldziher talked about the group that rejected it, and labelled them "orthodox" specifically because they rejected it.[49]

Scholars like Edward Grant continued to accept the "Orientalist" argument that Greek science in general, with what it owes to Aristotelian philosophy, was met with rebuttal by the Islamic "orthodoxy."[50] As Grant presents it, "[…] most Muslim theologians believed, on the basis of the Koran, that God caused everything directly and immediately and that natural things were incapable of acting directly on other natural things. Although secondary causation is usually assumed in scientific research, most Muslim theologians opposed it, fearing that the study of Greek philosophy and science would make their students hostile to religion."[51]

While many folk practices of medicine continued among the general population, Greek medicine, through the translation movement, came to be adapted, adopted, practiced and studied by Muslims in an academic context. Indeed, Greek medicine thrived because of its relative potency compared to folk practices, and because pre-Islamic pagan traditions were often conflicting with

[47] The most obvious problem with the term "orthodoxy" when referring to Islam is the absence of any official normalizing institution. Unlike the Catholic Christian's clergy, Muslims do not have a unique institutionalized establishment responsible for defining orthodoxy. Dimitri Gutas, *Greek Thought, Arabic Culture* (London: Routledge, 1998), 168.
[48] *Ibid.*
[49] *Ibid.*, 168.
[50] *Ibid*, 156-175;
[51] Edward Grant, *The Foundations of Modern Science in the Middle Ages: Their Religious, Institutional, and Intellectual Contexts* (Cambridge: Cambridge University Press, 1996), 178.

God's prescriptions.[52] Additional studies like that of Nahyan Fancy have shone light on this aspect of the historiography of the Islamic relationship with Greek science. Indeed, theologians who rejected Greek sciences "comprised only one group amongst the many, diverse theological and scholarly groups, all of whom were vying for the badge of 'orthodoxy.'"[53] Thus, since the critique of Goldziher by Gutas and the revisions of Sabra, it is generally accepted that Muslims of the 8th-9th centuries not only readily accepted the heritage of Greek sciences but actively sought it out.[54]

The Importance of Galen

A question remains: how did the science of Galen, a pagan, appeal to Muslims in such a way that it would, as Helena Paavilainen presents it, eclipse other pre-Islamic medical practices that were pagan as well?[55] Indeed, Galen was an active worshipper of Asclepius, and his polytheism was reflected in his works.[56] For example, Galen's commentary on the Hippocratic Oath contained "a major discussion on the role of pagan gods as founders and inspirers of medicine."[57]

Early Arab speaking Muslim scholars came into contact with the works of Galen through the 9th-century translations of Ḥunayn ibn Isḥāq, which tended to translate religiously offending

---

[52] Helena M. Paavilainen, *Medieval Pharmacotherapy, Continuity and Change: Case Studies from Ibn Sīnā and some of his Late Medieval Commentators* (Brill: Leiden, 2009), 16.
[53] Fancy, "Pulmonary Transit and Bodily Resurrection," 15.
[54] A. I. Sabra, "The Appropriation and Subsequent Naturalization of Greek Science in Medieval Islam: A Preliminary Statement," *History of Science* 25 (1987), 223-243.
[55] Paavilainen, *Medieval Pharmacotherapy*, 16-17.
[56] Fridolf Kudlien, "Galen's Religious Beliefs," in *Galen: Problems and Prospects*, edited by Vivian Nutton, (London: The Wellcome Institute for the History of Medicine, 1981), 117-127.
[57] Vivian Nutton, "God, Galen and the Depaganization of Ancient Medicine," in *Religion and Medicine in the Middle Ages*, eds. Peter Biller and Joseph Ziegler (Rochester, NY: York Medieval Press, 2001), 27.

words "by more neutral equivalents."[58] Thus, he treated Galen's gods as historical characters, spirits or angels, transformed sacrifices to Asclepius by sacrifices "to God *in the name of Asclepius,*"[59] and attributed medical cure "*to God through* [...] Asclepius."[60] In his commentaries of Galenic works as well, Ḥunayn explained "the deification of Asclepius in terms of the assimilation of Ascelpius's rational soul to the divine, which adorned it with all the virtues."[61] The Greek medical theory that Muslims had access to had thus been precedingly digested and at least somewhat adapted by the monotheist Syriac-Christian translators.

According to Vivian Nutton, the predominance of Galen's thought in the Muslim world can be explained though four main factors. First of all, Nutton notes that the period of late Antiquity was marked by a scarcity of books and intellectual institutions of quality. In this context, the abundance of material that the Galenic corpus represented and the cohesiveness of his medicine were appealing and almost miraculous.[62]

Secondly, Nutton stresses the strength of Galen's words. Indeed, "where his logic failed to point out the weakness in an opponent's case, and that was rare, his urgent rhetoric could convince his readers that his was the only true explanation."[63] Galen was a good orator, one of the best among those accessible.

Thirdly, Galen's medicine was anchored in the world described by Plato and Aristotle. It was informed by Plato's anatomy, physiology, and his idea of the soul as tripartite as well as Aristotle's physical world that included the principle of the four elements (fire, water, air, earth)

---

58 *Ibid.*
59 *Ibid.*
60 *Ibid.*
61 *Ibid.*
62 *Ibid.*, 23.
63 *Ibid.*

and the four qualities (hot, wet, cold, dry).[64] This world was dominated above all by purpose, and this teleology resonated with Islamic doctrine. Deriving the certainty of divinity from the purposefulness of creation, Galen attracted the interest of Muslim theologians as well as doctors. Galen's treatise *On the Usefulness of the Parts of the Body* is well known for its teleological position, and for being the first complete description of the anatomy of the human spine. He explains that every detail of the anatomy of animals are purposeful, and that "Nature" has created the parts of our bodies in a way that they have many uses at once. Thus, the spine has been made "like the keel of the body that is necessary for life," in a way that allows us to walk erect and allows each animal to walk in the posture that is the best for it. And likewise, "Nature" employs one construction for many uses at once, "so it is in this instance too; first she [Nature] scooped out the interior of all the vertebrae, preparing thus a suitable pathway for the portion of the encephalon that was to descend along it, and, secondly, she did not make the whole spine from one simple, uncompounded bone."[65] We shall discuss the principle of purposefulness in matters of medical philosophy further along, as well as the impacts of this principle on later medical theory, but let us note that teleology was an important factor that contributed to the success of Galen's work, and Greek science in general, in the Islamic context.

Galen's teleology did not merely support the certainty of the existence of God; it also suggested that through the knowledge of His creation, one could come to know God himself and His attributes, as well as glorify Him through His creation. Examining a passage where Niẓam al-Dīn al-Nīsābūrī (d. 1330) compared the principles (*uṣūl*) of jurisprudence (*fiqh*) to those of astronomy (*hayʾa*), Robert Morrison concluded that to partisans of natural theology, the study of

---

[64] *Ibid.*, 23-24.
[65] Galen, *Galen on the Usefulness of the Parts of the Body. De Usu Partium*, trans. Margaret Tallmadge May (Ithaca, NY: Cornell University Press, 1968), 507.

nature "enhanced one's appreciation of God's majesty and wisdom in creation."[66] Ḥājjī Khalīfa (d. 1657), in his *Kashf al-Ẓunūn*, an extensive bibliographical encyclopaedia of sciences, stated that no one who did not possess the knowledge of anatomy (*tashrīḥ*), along with that of astronomy, could claim to have knowledge of God.[67]

Galen's theology located divinity, be it God or gods, in the physical world, not outside of it. Far from a remote being, passive beyond the firmament, Asclepius had saved Galen more than once, and helped him cure his own medical affliction.[68] Differing from the nature of Judeo-Christian miracles, Galen's "demiurge" worked in his own creation and when he cures, it is through "scientifically" explicable ways.[69] To him, the epistemological nature and significance of the involvement of Asclepius in the healing processes, i.e. through the dream-advices that we discussed earlier, was that it should be expected to confirm the medical theory achieved by logic and theoretical thinking, it should "fit his own concepts and standards of rational medicine."[70]

Thus, while we can see that Greek medicine was often rid of references to pagan gods and beliefs by the translators, it managed to keep Galen's naturalistic conceptualisation of health and illness, as well as its teleological character, and could consequently resonate with a medical theory set in a monotheistic religious context. This compatibility was an important factor in the attitudes of Muslims toward him and the science that he represented.

---

[66] Robert Morrison, "Islamic Perspectives on Natural Theology," in *The Oxford Handbook of Natural Theology*, edited by John Hedley Brooke, Russel Re Manning, and Fraser Watts (Oxford: Oxford University Press, 2013), 156-157.
[67] Ḥājjī Khalīfa, *Kashf al-ẓunūn 'an asāmī al-kutub wa-al-funūn*, edited by Kilisli Muallim Rifat and Muhammad Sharaf al-Dīn Yāltaqāyā (Istanbul: Wakālat al-Ma'ārif, 1941-1943), 409.
[68] Galen, *De propriis placitis, On My Own Opinion*, ed. and trans. Vivian Nutton (Berlin: Akademie Verlag, 1999), 134-140.
[69] Richard Walzer, *Galen on Jews and Christians* (London: Oxford University Press, 1949), 23-37.
[70] Kudlien, "Galen's Religious Beliefs," 122-123.

The Intermediary Context and the Philosopher-Physician

The success and popularity of Galen in the Islamic context and throughout the Middle Ages may be explained by his prior success in late Antiquity in the main centers of intellectual activity. Unfortunately, due to the lack of sources, information is scarce about the medical tradition of the intermediary context between Galen in the 2nd-3rd centuries and the time of the translation movement. Certain Islamicate authors like Ḥunayn ibn Isḥāq described the medical learning that was dispensed in Alexandria. Toward the end of Antiquity, Alexandria had developed into one of the major places where medicine based on naturalistic and rational thinking was practiced and taught.[71] In the 4th century, the biographies of 23 sophists and philosophers of the last two centuries compiled by Eunapios (d. 5th c.), Greek sophist and historian, show how these scholars and their students gradually moved toward Alexandria.[72] The *Collectiones medicae* of Oribasius (d. 403), medical writer and personal physician of Roman emperor Julian the Apostate (d. 363), was an Alexandrian testimony of the growing influence of Galen.[73] According to Gotthard Strohmaier, the medicine that was practiced and taught in Alexandria acted as an intermediary between Galenic medicine and in a larger sense the Greek medical tradition and the Syrian-Arab tradition as well as the Byzantine tradition, and the developments that occurred there had influence on the practices of learning as far as Syria, and thus had influence on the later traditions as well.[74] Alexandria might not have been the only major center of medical learning, but the reason for our emphasis here is that the form that it took contributed in furthering the influence of Galen's works and to increasing

[71] Strohmaier, "Reception and Tradition," 143.
[72] Robert J. Penella., *Greek Philosophers and Sophists* (Leeds: Francis Cairn Ltd, 1990), 1-9.
[73] Strohmaier, "Reception and Tradition," 143.
[74] *Ibid.*, 145-147.

the prestige it enjoyed later, as shown by the standings of "l'éminent Galien"[75]in the translations of famous Islamicate authors like Yūḥannā ibn Māsawayh (d. 857) or Ḥunayn ibn Isḥāq.

There were two major tendencies in the evolution of medical knowledge in Alexandria. These tendencies further point to the pluralistic nature of the medical heritage that Muslims encountered. At one end of the spectrum, there existed a tendency to "summarize knowledge in the form of manuals designed for immediate practical application."[76] At the other end of the spectrum, there was also a tendency to emphasize theory over everything.[77] The theoretical orientation of the Alexandrian medical tradition is shown by the organization of learning in Alexandria as described by Ḥunayn ibn Isḥāq (d. 873) in his *Missive to ʿAlī Ibn Yaḥyỳ on Galen's Books* ("*Risālat Ḥunayn Ibn Isḥāq ilā ʿAlī ibn Yaḥyỳ fī dhikr mā turjima min kutub Jālīnūs bi-ʿilmih wa baʿḍ mā lam yutarjam*"), and that of Ibn Riḍwān in a dedicated chapter of his *Useful Book on the Quality of Medical Education.*[78] Indeed, this "curriculum" was composed originally of sixteen treatises of the Galenic corpus and four treatises of the Hippocratic corpus. The treatise that was generally taught first was *De Sectis ad eos qui introducuntur*, in which Galen presents his eclectic method and its superiority over other medical sects. Surely, another treatise would have been chosen as introductory material if medical practice was a priority.[79]

---

[75] Yūḥannā ibn Māsawayh, *Le Livre des Axiomes Médicaux (Aphorismi)*, trans. Danielle Jacquart and Gérard Troupeau (Genève: Librairie Droz, 1980), 222.
[76] *Ibid.*, 143.
[77] As an example of this theoretically oriented inclination, Strohmaier points to the Alexandrian physician Magnus whose skills in theoretical debates were so great that he could prove that a patient of another physician was still sick without seeing him. *Ibid.*, 144. See also Penella, *Greek Philosophers and Sophists*, 115-117.
[78] A. Z. Iskandar "An Attempted Reconstruction of the Late Alexandrian Curriculum," *Medical History* 20 (1976), 236-237.
[79] Strohmaier, "Reception and Tradition," 144; Iskandar, "An Attempted Reconstruction," 238-239.

Rationalism in the practice and the theory of medicine came hand in hand with Galen's emphasis on the importance for the doctor to also be a philosopher. The philosopher-physician, as an ideal of Greek medicine, avoids grief and knows the difference between good and bad habits; he cultivates virtues such as temperance, wisdom, courage.[80] In his practice of healing others and in his search for knowledge, he values sobriety, humility, perseverance; he does not pass judgment unknowingly, but shows empathy.[81] Furthermore, before even starting to study medicine proper and in accord with what Strohmaier and Iskandar described as the "curriculum" of the "School of Alexandria", the philosopher-physician should be trained in the arts of "logic, physics, arithmetic, numerals, measurement, geometry, the compounding of drugs, astrology, and ethics."[82] Thusly, the study of these subject prepares the student's intellect, introduces him to the demonstrative method, and "fosters the love of truth."[83] In his *al-Nāfiʿ fī kayfiyyat taʿlīm ṣināʿat al-ṭibb* (Useful Book on the Manner of Medical Education), Ibn Riḍwān uses Galen's book *That the Excellent Physician is a Philosopher* as a model to describe the preferable path of the studies of an aspiring doctor.[84] Galen's theory of the philosopher-physician was thus not just a guide to medical education but also a witness to the ideas of a good scholar and a good person, and thus resonated with Islamic values.

One may not approach the subject of ethics in the profession of the physician without mentioning the famed *Hippocratic Oath*. The *Oath* presented ethical concerns about the possible issues of medical practice and the responsibilities of a practitioner that resonated with Islamic ethical prescriptions. Indeed, the themes of the *Oath* revolved around the obligation not to cause

[80] Vivian Nutton, "God, Galen and the Depaganization of Ancient Medicine", 23.
[81] Iskandar, "An Attempted Reconstruction", 235-258.
[82] *Ibid.*, 257.
[83] Ibid.
[84] *Ibid.* 239-241.

harm, nor to prevent the conception of children, to practice the profession in a pure and holy way, and not to abuse the medical profession in his interactions with men and women, etc.[85] The survival of the *Oath* and its passage into Arab hands is attested mainly by Ḥunayn's translation of an ancient commentary of the *Oath* into Syriac and the subsequent translation into Arabic by Ḥunayn's nephew Ḥubaysh ibn al-Ḥasan al-Dimashqī (fl. second half of the 9th century).[86] As also occurred in the Christian West,[87] the *Oath* was also adapted by Islamicate doctors in order to provide a baseline for the ethics of the doctor.

Medical Ethics and the *Oath* of Hippocrates

One of the means through which the profession of physician was kept in check was the office of *ḥisba* ("commanding right and forbidding wrong"). How much of the actions of the *muḥtassib* (the officer of *ḥisba*) actually impacted the work of physicians is obviously a very difficult question to answer, but the literature produced in order to guide these officers may be indicative of the role they played, and the sensibilities of Muslims concerning medicine. As is shown in some of the manuals of *ḥisba* that have survived, it was among the responsibilities of the *muḥtassib* to require all physicians to take the *Hippocratic Oath* (*ʿahd Buqrāṭ*) and

> "[...] swear not to administer harmful medicine to anyone, not to prepare poison for them, not to describe amulets to anyone from the general public, not to mention to women the medicine used for abortions and not to mention to men the medicine preventing the

[85] Steven H. Miles, *The Hippocratic Oath*, 49-159.
[86] Franz Rosenthal, "An Ancient Commentary on the Hippocratic Oath," *Bulletin of the History of Medicine* 30 (1956): 81-87.
[87] Owsei Temkin, *Hippocrates in a World of Pagans and Christians* (Baltimore: The Johns Hopkins University Press, 1991), 183.

begetting of children. They must avert their eyes from the women's quarters when they visit their patients, and they must not disclose secrets nor lift up the veils."[88]

The adoption of the *Oath* by officers of *ḥisba* represents the first time in history that a version of the *Oath* was used by a state authority.[89] ʿAbd al-Raḥmān ibn Nasr al-Shayzarī's (d. 1193) manual of *ḥisba*, titled *Nihāyat al-rutba fī ṭalab al-ḥisba* (*The Utmost Authority in the Pursuit of Ḥisba)* presents many details on the context of the practice of medicine. Aside from taking the *Oath*, the physician must be examined on the basis of Ḥunayn ibn Isḥāq's *The Trial of the Physician*[90] and certain specialists must be knowledgeable in the most popular books that pertain to their expertise. Thus, the eye-doctors must be tested on *The Ten Treatises of the Eye* of Ḥunayn; the bone setters must have mastered the *De Medica Syntagma* (*Thesaurus on Medicine*) of Paul of Aegina (d. 690); and the surgeons should know the *Kata Genos* of Galen.[91]

The work of al-Shayzarī enjoyed a great contemporary significance for it was the first extant book on the practical application of *ḥisba* and its content was further used by later authors of guides for the *muḥtassib*. This is the case of Ibn al-Ukhuwwa (d. 1338), an Egyptian shāfiʿī scholar, and Ibn Bassām (fl. 14th c.), who took up al-Shayzarī's work almost word for word, and even copied the order of the chapters, all while expanding the content.[92]

[88] ʿAbd al-Raḥmān ibn Nasr al-Shayzarī, *The Book of the Islamic Market Inspector: Nihāyat al-Rutba fī Ṭalab al-Ḥisba (The Utmost Authority in the Pursuit of Ḥisba)*, trans. R. P. Buckley (Oxford: Oxford University Press, 1999), 115.
[89] Strohmaier, "Reception and Tradition," 156.
[90] Ibn al-Nadīm, *The Fihrist*, 693-694.
[91] al-Shayzarī, *The Book of the Islamic Market Inspector*, 116-118.
[92] *Ibid.*, 1-15.

Ibn Sīnā's Canon of Medicine

The Greek ethical and educational context of the practice and the learning of the art of medicine came to be quite influential on medicine in the Islamic context. In terms of medical theory as well, the authors of medical literature inherited the ideas of Hippocrates, Aristotle and Galen.

Determining what the authors of Prophetic Medicine of the 13th-14th centuries had effectively read of the medical literature circulating in the Muslim world could be the object of a separate research of its own. However, one work of medicine seems impossible to omit when trying to paint the context of the medical literature after the 11th century: the famed *Canon of Medicine* (*al-Qānūn fī al-Ṭibb*) of Ibn Sīnā, or Avicenna (d. 1037). In its essentials, the medical work of Ibn Sīnā did not differ much from that of his celebrated predecessors such as al-Rāzī (d. 920). Indeed, both had presented the doctrines of Hippocrates modified and informed by the work of Aristotle and Galen. Ibn Sīnā's achievement, however, consisted in a higher degree of systematization and a comprehensiveness unequaled in his age.[93] I will therefore attempt to summarize some of the main principles of Avicennian medicine in order to give a sense of the medical theory which may have informed the authors of Prophetic Medicine.

Causation in in the *Canon* is explained through Aristotelian philosophy. The understanding of the four causes is necessary to acquire knowledge of something: the "material" cause, or what the thing is made of; the "efficient" cause, or that which molds it; the "formal" cause or that which determines its shape and quality; and the "final" cause, or the function for which it is made.[94]

---

[93] Avicenna, *The General Principles of Avicenna's Canon of Medicine*, trans. Mazhar H. Shah (Karachi: Naveed Clinic, 1966), iii.
[94] *Ibid.*, 19.

Avicennian medicine makes use of Aristotelian causes because "the knowledge of a material object can only be obtained by determining its origin and causes [...]."[95]The application of these principles in medicine allows for approaching illness as a product of: "(a) inheritance–the stuff or material [the person] is made of; (b) the kind of temperament, structure and strength of faculties [the person] has; (c) the type of factors operating on [the person] from outside; and (d) [the] nature's own attempt at the maintenance of [a person's] life functions."[96]

In "Nature of Man", Hippocrates had attempted to reconcile Empedocles' (d. 448 BCE) materialism, according to which all material bodies were made of a combination of fire, air, water and earth, and Plato's (d. 400 BCE) idealism, which explains that matter does not have any real existence, except in the human mind. As a result, and as explained in the *Canon of Medicine*, the concept of elements in the sense of basic "fixed and unalterable entities" is shifted to the four primary qualities (*quwā*), i.e. heat, cold, moisture and dryness. Thus, the substances which were previously known as *elements* (fire, air, water and earth) are also compounded of primary qualities, but stand as a symbol of the exclusive dominance of one of the primary qualities.[97]

Following our brief overview of causation and elements in Avicennian medical theory, let us present also the Canon's use of "temperaments" (*mizāj*). Temperament corresponds to "the pattern of activity and reactivity of the body [or its parts] expressed in the terms of elementary qualities (*quwā*) namely heat, cold, dryness and moisture."[98] This pattern rests at the core of the humoral theory as developed by the Greeks and adopted by the Arabs, because it can exhibit one

---

95 *Ibid.*
96 *Ibid.*, xiii.
97 *Ibid.*, xiii-xiv.
98 *Ibid.*, xix.

of two states: balance (*muʿtadil*) and imbalance (*kharij ʿan al-ʿitidal*).[99] As an allopathic system of medicine, the medical theory of Ibn Sīnā rates the intensity of the qualities of medicaments and uses a drug of a certain quality to resolve a condition of the opposite quality.[100]

As for the "humors" (*akhlāṭ*), Hippocrates was the first to observe and distinguish the blood humor, the phlegm, the yellow bile and the black bile. In time, Galen, following Hippocrates in his *Nature of Man*[101], would theorize that all diseases were the effect of imbalance, i.e. irregular distribution, of the humors.[102] In the Canon, "the dominance of each humor is recognized from its characteristic colour and qualities and from the age and temperament of the patient, nature of food, tempo of activity and the prevailing season."[103]

Avicennian medical theory is rounded up by the principle of *faculties*. The *physical faculty* (*ṭabīʿiyya*) serves the body for its nutrition and its growth; its center is the liver. The *nervous faculty* (*nafsāniyya*) is responsible for sensation and movement; its center is the brain. The *vital faculty* (*ḥaywāniyya*) is responsible for life and the activity of organs and tissue, and its center is the heart.[104]

Authors of Prophetic Medicine such as Ibn Qayyīm al-Jawziyya (d. 1350) were theologians and philosophers and they were often accomplished practising physicians. As such, it is not surprising to find that the sections of medical theory included in their works on the medicine of the Prophet shared the same foundations.[105] It was not rare to find direct references to Ibn Sīnā's

---

99 Balance is not meant here as *equality*, for it is not referred to as the quantitative proportion of the primary qualities, but rather a proportion that results in a 'normal' functioning of the body or its parts. *Ibid.*, 24-25.
100 *Ibid.*, xx-xxi.
101 Jouanna, *Greek Medicine from Hippocrates to Galen: Selected Papers* (Leiden: Brill, 2012), 310-359.
102 *Ibid.*, xxiv.
103 *Ibid.*, xxv.
104 Avicenna, *The General Principles*, 125-137.
105 Ibn Qayyīm al-Jawziyya, *Medicine of the Prophet*, xiii.

opinions, and even to those of Galen and Hippocrates. in the works of many authors of Prophetic Medicine, in their section on medical theory, these opinions were then supported by sayings of the Prophet or of his Companions or by the Qur'an.[106]

These works did not limit themselves to medical theory. In fact, the bulk of the treatises, especially the later ones, consisted in a compendium of foodstuff and simple drugs, along with the diseases that they should help cure, and sometimes with their natural qualities (hot, cold, dry or moist). In the same way, the content of these parts of the treatises mostly included plants and foodstuff as they were earlier recorded by Dioscorides (d. 90 CE) in his *De Materia Medica*[107] and included some additions that were made by medieval pharmacologists.[108]

The impact of the evolution of Greek medicine on medicine in Islam and, by extension Prophetic Medicine, is undeniable. Both directly and indirectly, the ideas and ideals of influential Greek physicians and medical writers came to be of first importance to the authors of this genre. One could argue that the "medicine of the prophet" was indeed given an ironic name, for it was basically made up of medical theory and pharmacology taken almost straight from the Greeks. Aside from the obvious borrowing in terms of content, we must understand that the relationship between medicine and religion in the Greek context contributed to making medicine what it was when the Arabs started translating the works of the Ancients. The way medicine and philosophy was shaped by their Greek origins and evolution culminated in the medical corpus and the epistemological views on medicine that the Arabs took up.

---

[106] Perho, *The Prophet's Medicine*, 78-79.

[107] Dioscorides Pedanius of Anazarbos, *De Materia Medica*, trans. Lily Y. Beck (Hildesheim: Olms-Weidmann, 2005).

[108] Micheal Dols, *Medieval Islamic Medicine: Ibn Riḍwān's treatise, "On the Prevention of Bodily Ills in Egypt,"* (Berkeley: University of California Press, 1984), 15.

CHAPTER 2: THE POLITICAL, INTELLECTUAL AND RELIGIOUS CONTEXTS OF EARLY MAMLŪK CAIRO AND DAMASCUS

The study of the history of science in the Islamic context has in the past had to deal with, and overcome, the assumption of the irrationality of Islam and its incompatibility with reason as well as with the Greek knowledge traditions the Muslims world inherited. This point of view, along with all that resulted from it, stems from the post-enlightenment idea that reason and religious revelation are intrinsically hostile toward one another. As we have seen earlier, such an assumption gave rise to what are referred to as the "marginality" thesis, which assumes that rational Islamic science was marginalized because of the absence of institutional support, and the "warfare" thesis, according to which it was directly attacked. Our focus on context, in the previous chapter and the present one, stems from the nature of modern historiography of Islamic science.

Recently, revisionist authors have worked to debunk the conception of Islamic science that was too dependant on the premise of the incompatible nature of reason and religion. These authors also criticized the belief that Islamic science was merely Greek science in Arabic, by providing evidence of developments in mathematics, astronomy, optics, medicine, etc., and by confronting the traditional periodization of the "Decline of Islamic Science", or challenging its existence altogether.[109]

[109] For a revision of the old historiography of Islamic science, see particularly A.I. Sabra, "The Appropriation and Subsequent." For a survey of the developments brought about in Islamic science, see Roshdi Rashed (ed.), *Encyclopedia of the History of Arabic Science*, 3 vols. (London: Routlege, 1996). For a challenging look at the periodization of the "Decline of Islamic Science", see George Saliba, "Seeking the Origins of Modern Science?" *Bulletin of the Royal Institute of Inter-Faith Studies* 1 (1999): 139-152; George Saliba, *A History of Arabic Astronomy:*

Certain scholars have even more recently made attempts to provide a critical look into the works that originated from this historiographical shift and have participated in illustrating some of their limitations. This is the case of Nahyan Fancy's dissertation "Pulmonary Transit and Bodily Resurrection," which criticizes some changes brought about in the study of Islamic sciences by the revisionist authors like Roshdi Rashed, George Saliba and A. I. Sabra. Among these limitations, Fancy mentions the relative lack of studies dedicated to medicine in Islam in the revisionist historiography.[110] Irmeli Perho's 1995 study of Prophetic Medicine is the first study of Prophetic Medicine with a revisionist point of view, but it exhibits another one of the limitations of the new historiography. Nahyan Fancy states that "historians are still primarily interested in determining how a certain Islamic medical tract relates to its Greek predecessor,"[111] something we have pointed to previously. The past decades have seen the exemplary works of authors who tried to locate Islamic medicine in its context, but these are still uncommon.[112] And indeed, Perho's work is a critique of earlier works on Prophetic Medicine like that of Manfred Ullmann[113] and Christoph Bürgel[114], but it still stems from the same model of studying Islamic Sciences by comparing Islamic authors to their Greek predecessors. While attempting to present some of the context of its development, Perho's question on Prophetic Medicine remains along the lines of the early revisionists' investigations, and shares their limitations: "What parts of Hippocrates', Galen's and Avicenna's legacy can we find in Prophetic Medicine?" These are questions that we cannot

---

Planetary Theories During the Golden Age of Islam (New York: New York University Press, 1994); and Jamil Ragep, "Freeing Astronomy from Philosophy: An Aspect of Islamic Influence on Science," *Osiris* 16 (2001): 49-71.

[110] This under-representation can be perceived in Rashed, *Encyclopedia*; and in J. Hogendijk and A. I. Sabra, *The Enterprise of Science in Islam: New Perspectives* (Cambridge: MIT Press, 2003). Both works include merely one article on medicine. Fancy, "Pulmonary Transit and Bodily Resurrection," 20-21.

[111] Fancy, "Pulmonary Transit and Bodily Resurrection," 20-21.

[112] For examples, see Michael Dols, *The Black Death in the Middle East* (Princeton: Princeton University Press, 1977); and *Majnūn: The Madmen in the Medieval Islamic World* (Oxford: Clarendon Press, 1992); and Emily Savage-Smith, "The Practice of Surgery in Islamic Lands: Myth and Reality," *History of Medicine* 13 (2000): 307-321.

[113] Manfred Ullmann, *Die Medizin im Islam* (Leiden: Handbuch der Orientalistik, 1970).

[114] Bürgel, "Secular and Religious Features".

deem pointless, but approaching the subject in this framework might limit our understanding of the socio-political, economic and historical circumstances that surrounded it.

Another problem with the recent study of Arab sciences concerns the framework of the inevitable dichotomy of purposes and methods between the "scientific" on one side, i.e. driven by the experimental method of observation, theory, and reproducibility, and the "unscientific" on the other side, i.e. personal or theological purposes and methods. Dimitri Gutas' model for studying the history of science, described in his article "Certainty, Doubts and Error: Comments on the Epistemological Foundations of Medieval Arabic Science" might constrain our understanding of Islamic science to distinctions of the "scientific" merits versus the "unscientific" merits of the Arab scholars' works.[115]

Other scholars instead propose that historians of science abandon this dichotomy of a universal criterion in favor of considering "what the historical actors themselves considered scientific and non-scientific."[116] As stated earlier, my goal in this study of Prophetic Medicine is to provide an outlook of the genre while avoiding universal qualifications of scientific and unscientific, and to shed light on the multi-faceted aspects of Prophetic Medicine while keeping the context of the authors in mind. To this end, I will examine the political, intellectual and religious context of the lives of the scholars who participated in the development of this genre.

[115] Dimitri Gutas, "Certainty, Doubt, Error: Comments on the Epistemological Foundations of Medieval Arabic Science," *Early Science and Medicine* 7 (2002): 287.
[116] Fancy, "Pulmonary Transit and Bodily Resurrection," 23-24.

Political Context of late Seljūq and Early Mamlūk Cairo and Damascus

The context under the late Seljūqs and the early Mamlūks was crucial to the evolution of Prophetic Medicine for two main reasons: first, in search of legitimization, the rulers sought to appear as upholders of the faith and defenders of the religious establishment, and one way by which they manifested this support was by providing an essential space for a number of groups, including "traditionalists". Second, the *ʿulamāʾ* (religious scholars) were not necessarily satisfied with the ethnic background and the behaviours of the ruling elite; their practices, to some, presented incompatibilities with religious doctrine, and prompted the sentiment that a return to a more "original" version of Islam was imperative.

In the 12th century, there occurred the first major military setbacks in the Islamic world: the Christian Crusades in Syria and the *Reconquista* in Spain. The European advance is stopped in Syria by the reunification of most of Syria and Egypt under the leadership of Saladin (d. 1193).

The 13th century brings the Mongol invasions in the Eastern portions of the Islamic world. In 1258, Baghdad, capital of the ʿAbbāsid caliphate, is taken by the invaders. The advance of the Mongols was stopped by the new Mamlūk Sultanate of Cairo under Baybars al-Bunduqdārī (d. 1277). In 1250, the last Ayyūbid sultan dies and one of the main difficulties of the Mamlūk system is exacerbated: while the slave-soldiers were generally loyal to their master, the ruler seldom managed to transfer this loyalty to his heir. The ruling elite was made up of purchased slaves that had climbed through the military ranks. The descendants of these Mamlūks, the members of the *awlād al-nās*, were free-born Muslims and were consequently kept out of the higher offices of the military hierarchy. Higher positions were exclusively given to purchased Mamlūks, the only exception being the sultanate itself.[117] One of the alternative career paths pursued by their sons was that of scholars, which allowed them to assimilate into the non-Mamlūk society. This was the case of chroniclers like Ibn al-Dawādārī (fl. 1335), Ibn Taghrībirdī (d. 1470) and Ibn Ṭūlūn (d. 1546).[118]

The Vibrant Intellectual Activity of the 11th to 13th Centuries

Since the beginnings of Islam, and especially since the ʾUmayyad califate, Damascus had assumed a very prominent position in the Islamic world as a cultural center. As explained in Joan E. Gilbert's "Institutionalization of Muslim-Scholarship and Professionalization of Ulama in Medieval Damascus," Damascus in the early centuries of Islam was one of the most prominent epicenters of an "international system of Muslim scholarship" characterized by the wide movements of scholars for the purpose of learning and teaching.[119] This "system" went from "regularized practices" to an "institutionalized system" during the late 11th to the 13th centuries. To Gilbert, the "Damascus-Cairo axis" of professional pursuit in the Muslim world played a major role in the institutionalization of scholarly activities, where "institutionalization meant permanent provision of special places of instruction, residence, and employment for a majority of scholars and lasting endowments to pay the salaries of the personnel and building costs."[120] The construction, between the second half of the 11th and the end of the 13th centuries, of dozens of

---

[117] Between 1250 and 1382, as many as seventeen sultans were members of the *awlād al-nās*, while only seven were purchased Mamlūks. P. M. Holt, *The Age of the Crusades: The Near East from the Eleventh Century to 1517* (London: Longman, 1986), 141.
[118] *Ibid.*, 140-141.
[119] Joan E. Gilbert, "Institutionalization of Muslim-Scholarship and Professionalization of Ulama in Medieval Damascus," *Studia Islamica* 52 (1980): 105-112.
[120] *Ibid.*, 114.

religious establishments, such as *madrasas* along with *dar al-ḥadīth*s and places of *ṣūfī* education, represented the material requirement for the institutionalization that took place. These establishments created hundreds of relatively permanent employment positions for scholars, of local and foreign origin, thus professionalizing the occupation of the *'ulama'*.[121]

The Seljūqs were the first to attempt to associate their state government with the religious elite through support of the *madrasa*s, and promoting the cause of a "*Sunnī* revival", which we shall discuss later. According to Carla L. Klausner, "[…] the early organizers of the empire hoped in this way to […] secure the support of the religious classes by giving them a stake in the proper functioning of the state, and to bolster the civil administration against the expected encroachments of the military establishment."[122]

According to A. I. Sabra, the Greek sciences, along with their theories in cosmology, metaphysics and epistemology, gradually made their way in these establishments of learning, as is shown by the wide-ranging translation movement that occurred and the naturalization that followed it.[123] To Sabra, alternatives were developed in the *madrasa*, and there emerged "a homegrown religious philosophy" claiming to challenge the Greek paradigms.[124] The *madrasas* were originally conceived as schools of Islamic law, but the private character of the endowments that instituted them allowed for a greater degree of informality and a considerable variety of intellectual pursuits depending on local circumstances and interests of professors and patrons. While Islamic law continued to be the prime subject of studies in the *madrasa*, many of them

---

[121] *Ibid.*, 113-126.
[122] Carla L. Klausner. *The Seljuk Vezirate: A Study of Civil Administration 1055-1194* (Cambridge: Harvard University Press, 1973), 22.
[123] A. I. Sabra, "Situating Arabic Science: Locality versus Essence," *Isis* 87 (1996): 664-665.
[124] A. I. Sabra, "The Appropriation and Subsequent Naturalization of Greek Science in Medieval Islam: A Preliminary Statement," *History of Science* 25 (1987): 223-243.

included arithmetic, algebra, astronomy, logic, linguistics, and rhetoric. These originally "secular" sciences were taken as introductory material to prepare the jurist to the study of law in the madrasas.[125]

The role of Damascus as a cultural center was enlivened in the 13th c. by the affluence of refugees coming from the fringes of Islamic lands. Many of these refugees were from the elite, intellectuals of all sorts and members of the *ʿulamāʾ*. The events that shook the 13th century contributed in increasing the affluence of scholars in the centers of high learning of Syria and Egypt, bringing together people who themselves brought along many rival intellectual and religious positions.[126]

The refugees were not only Muslims: the global historical context of the time conditioned an affluence of non-Muslim elites in cities, as well as in the profession of medicine. Indeed, the cohesion of the eastern Islamic world was shattered by the Mongol invasion: the invaders provoked a westward movement of population that made many non-Muslims settle down in the main urban centers of Syria and Egypt. According to Perho, it is precisely these circumstances that pressed certain *ḥadīth* scholars to show interest in Galenic medicine and to create the genre of Prophetic Medicine in an attempt to introduce more Muslims to the medical arts.[127]

Muslim and *dhimmī* populations sometimes clashed, which led to riots, and sometimes to the creation and upholding of laws of discriminatory nature against non-Muslims, especially for the acquisition of offices of bureaucracy. Al-Maqrīzī (d. 1442) reports that following anti-*dhimmīs*

---

125 *Ibid.*
126 Nahyan A.G. Fancy, *Science and Religion in Mamluk Egypt: Ibn al-Nafīs, Pulmonary Transit and Bodily Resurrection* (London and New York: Routledge, 2013), 16-17.
127 Perho, *The Prophet's Medicine*, 76-84.

riots in 1354 in Cairo, the *dhimmīs* were forbidden to practise medicine.[128] This might have been symptomatic of a growing presence of Muslims in the medical professions, because these *dhimmīs* had to be replaced with Muslims in order to provide the services of a physician to those that needed them. And these were needed indeed: Shāfiʿī scholar Taqī al-Dīn al-Subkī (d. 1355) had criticized the Mamlūk *amīrs* for employing physicians in all their fortresses, and for having physicians escort them on their travels, while they did not give the same favours to jurists.[129]

Not only did patronage from the Seljūq and Mamlūk elite help foster intellectual activity, the Mamlūk Sultanate's political system itself aided in the bourgeoning of many intellectual and religious institutions, which provided the physical context for the blooming of scholarly activity. Because the Sultan was not allowed to appoint his descendant as successor and because high offices were not necessarily hereditary, the military elite was constantly involved in power struggles which often culminated in the ruin of a family. Securing wealth and power was thus made arduous for elite households.[130]

According to Michael Chamberlain, who studied social practices of the 13th and 14th centuries in Damascus as well as the relationship between these practices and science, education and knowledge in general, there were three main reasons for the "disjunction in the long-term control of property"[131] and in the control of status of the lords of Damascus. Firstly, upon the death of a wealthy head of family, the division of property among a large number of heirs, was obligatory

---

128 *Ibid.*, 28.
129 Taqī al-Dīn ʿAlī ibn ʿAbd al-Kāfī al-Subkī, *The Restorer of Favours and the Restrainer of Chastisements: The Arabic Text with an Introduction and Notes* (London: Luzac, 1908), 34.
130 *Ibid.*
131 Micheal Chamberlain, *Knowledge and Social Practice in Medieval Damascus, 1190-1350* (Cambridge: Cambridge University Press, 1994), 27.

according to Islamic inheritance laws.[132] Property could thus hardly be kept intact and streamlined through a descent group.

Secondly, the structure of authority in families made it such that power was held by the senior male members of the *extended* family, instead of limited to a single line of descent within it. Property could not keep its integrity under the control of a single line of descent, and it was partitioned further by every generation.[133]

Thirdly, there were no "intermediate social structures such as formal estates or corporate bodies between the ruling groups and the general population."[134] As an effect, the households of lords of Damascus "could not reliably turn corporate social practices or entities to their benefit."[135]

To secure their wealth and maintain the sources of income into their households, families would take advantage of the Islamic religious endowments (*waqf*), thus creating several institutions that were more enduring than political power. The *waqf* could not be usurped, so the contract of its institution would often secure a supervisory office for a member of the ruling family, and it guaranteed the integrity of the wealth of a family through time and stability despite urban power struggles.[136]

The most common of the institutions established through *waqf* were *madrasas* (schools of law), which benefited the *ʿulamāʾ*, but also *bīmāristāns* (hospitals) and Ṣūfī establishments. In this manner, the military elite managed to obtain valuable support from the intellectual and religious elite, thus securing the military elite's economic future. In exchange, intellectual and religious

---

132 Joseph Schacht, *An Introduction to Islamic Law* (Oxford: Clarendon Press, 1982), 169-174.
133 Chamberlain, *Knowledge and Social Practice*, 28.
134 *Ibid.*
135 *Ibid.*
136 Fancy, *Science and Religion in Mamluk Egypt*, 17-18.

elites were supported by the rulers and their discourse benefitted from that much more attention. Chamberlain's strict definition of the *waqf* is the "immobilization of property for religious ends,"[137] and indeed most institutions created through waqf endowments were schools of Islamic law, which provided a spotlight and gave prominence to members of an intellectual elite interested in discussing and defining religious correctness. Under the Turkish Mamlūks (1250-1382), up to 74 teaching institutions were endowed or constructed in Cairo, and 30 in Damascus.[138]

The creation of intellectual institutions helped the ruling elite of the Mamlūk society advance their political goals, and the *waqf* helped them rigidify their economic and political assets. While they might have been relatively secondary, there were other reasons for supporting religious scholarship, as has been discussed by Jonathan Berkey. In theory, at least, every Mamlūk was exposed, during his training, to some basic concepts of religious practice and learning in Islam.

According to the account of famous historian al-Maqrīzī (d. 1442), the fundamentals of the Qur'ān, as well as the Arabic language, was taught to the young slave-soldiers by local Muslim scholars, along with the rituals of religion and some jurisprudence.[139] While many religious scholars and historians have been hostile toward the ethical leniency of the Mamlūks, Jonathan Berkey reminds us, as did Ulrich Haarmann before him[140], that "a large number of adult Mamlūks participated in the religious life of the Egyptian capital" and that their reported aversion for culture "should not obscure their eagerness to involve themselves in the transmission of Muslim learning."[141] Many of the young Mamlūks must have been influenced by their schooling and must

---

[137] Chamberlain, *Knowledge and Social Practice*, 51.
[138] Jonathan Berkey, *The Transmission of Knowledge in Medieval Cairo: A Social History of Islamic Education* (Princeton: Princeton University Press, 1992), 128-129.
[139] *Ibid.*, 147.
[140] Ulrich Haarmann, "Arabic in Speech, Turkish in Lineage: Mamluks and their Sons in the Intellectual Life of Fourteenth-Century Egypt and Syria," *Journal of Semitic Studies* 33 (1988): 81-86.
[141] Berkey, *The Transmission of Knowledge*, 147.

have felt that promoting Islamic scholarship allowed them to fulfill their duties as Muslims while maintaining their hold on the secular sphere.

Other less pious reasons for the promotion of such institutions might have been that endowed religious establishments concretely perpetuated the name of the donor's name. When a member of the elite endowed a *madrasa*, it would take his name. In a context of ferocious political competition, legitimacy of power over people and resources was a contested matter, and endowing a religious institution might have been a means of attaching prestige to one's name. This "symbolic capital", as Berkey presents it, was produced by the linking of the names of Mamlūks to some of the institutions that represented the most dignity in a society that valued culture and its transmission.[142]

In 1265, when Sultan Baybars accorded the office of chief judge to one of each of the four *Sunnī madhhabs*, he did so with the intent to accommodate the growing heterogeneity of the population.[143] However, there is little doubt that the Mamlūk rulers also recognized "the advantages that the gratitude and loyalty of an expanded judiciary and professoriate" could provide.[144] And as Joseph Escovitz demonstrated, the chroniclers mentioned many instances where they did indeed profit from the pressure they could exert on judges to vie in their favor.[145]

Thus, more often than not, the apparent piety of the policies of the Mamlūks covered an enduring attempt to cope for the lack of legitimacy of the rule of foreign slave-soldiers over their Muslim subjects and over an intellectual and religious elite that saw itself as rightful inheritors of

---

[142] *Ibid.*, 133-134.
[143] Joseph H. Escovitz, "The Establishment of Four Chief Judgeships in the Mamlūk Empire," *Journal of the American Oriental Society* 102 (1982): 529-531.
[144] *Ibid.*, Little, "Religion Under the Mamlūks," 174.
[145] Joseph H. Escovitz, "The Office of Qāḍī al-Quḍāt in Cairo under the Baḥrī Mamlūks" (Phd diss., McGill University, 1978), 148-158.

the culture and tradition of Islam. These policies did not end up safeguarding them from the skepticism of many members of the *'ulamā'*, as we have seen with the earlier example from al-Subkī, who, while mentioning the status enjoyed by physicians beside the *amīrs*, deplored that they did not employ Muslim jurists to inform them on religious matters.[146]

Contemporary historians painted an image of their rulers as "wild, ethically lax and only superficially Islamicized."[147] Ulrich Haarmann's study of the way the Arabs perceived the Turks provides one of the most sensible approaches to the conflicting and paradoxical relationships between the Arabs and their Mamlūk rulers. In this article, Haarmann explains that while the military exploits of the Mamlūks against the Crusaders and the Mongols enhanced their religious prestige, the positive assessment of their piety was a minority opinion among the chroniclers. The commonly circulated stereotype among the *'ulamā'* who were critical of the Mamlūks was that of the "villain, brutal, bloodthirsty and cunning"[148] barbarian, uninterested in culture, and even naturally incapable of it.

In the realm of scholarship as well, the members of the *awlād al-nās*, descendants of these "crude brutes," inherited the negative prejudice that Arabs scholars applied to their fathers. This translated in their case in the belittlement of their work.[149]

Certain scholars praised the rulers of Turkish origin. Ibn Khaldūn lauded the Mamlūks' nomadic virtues and the inflexibility of their religion, and Abū Ḥāmid al-Qudsī (d. 1483) admired

---

[146] al-Subkī, *The Restorer of Favours*, 34.
[147] Berkey, The Transmission of Knowledge, 144.
[148] Ulrich Haarmann, "Ideology and History, Identity and Alterity: The Arab Image of the Turks from the Abbasids to Modern Egypt," *International Journal of Middle East Studies* 20 (1988): 182-183.
[149] William Popper, "Sakhāwī's Criticism of Ibn Tāghrī Birdī," *Studi Orientalistici in Onore di Giorgio Levi della Vida*, vol. 3 (Rome: Instituto per l'Oriente, 1956), 388.

their "honesty, incorruptibility and spirit of sacrifice."[150] However, this attested to a situation that did not benefit everyone, and the majority of the contemporary chroniclers criticized their rulers, especially the scholars of Islam. The responsibility of the defense of Muslim beliefs and culture was shifting from the *ʿulamāʾ* to these foreign rulers.[151]

The centuries that marked the most important developments of Prophetic Medicine – which we will describe in the chapter 3 – were characterized by a very complex relationship between the intellectual and religious elites on the one side, and the military rulers on the other. These intellectuals were provided an important place in the public sphere due to different policies and practices of the Mamlūk elite, and their discourses sometimes became critical of the very establishment that allowed them to bloom.

Religious Traditionalism

In a context of a heightened convergence of elites in prominent urban areas and an increase in intellectual and religious activity, the "contest over correct belief was one of the premiere forms of social combat."[152] However, in Mamlūk society, there were no state or corporate bodies responsible for promulgating correct doctrine. The population of Damascus and Cairo was made up of *Shīʿīs*, *Sunnīs*, *Ṣūfīs*, philosophers, practitioners of *kalām*, etc. According to Chamberlain, there always remained an implicit disagreement concerning correct belief and thus an inherent

---

[150] *Ibid.*
[151] Haarmann, "Ideology and History", 182-183.
[152] Chamberlain, *Knowledge and Social Practice*, 167.

rivalry over the definition of orthodoxy. In general, however, they managed to keep their interactions peaceable and "rarely coerced others to abandon their beliefs."[153]

Under the Baḥrī Mamlūks (1250-1382), Damascus became the second capital of the realm and the administrative center of Syria, boasting an intense public life. Visiting Sultans, parading armies, as well as "sports displays, collective prayers and official receptions for rewarding officials [and] celebration of victories [...] brought masses of Sufis, jurists, students, and commoners into the streets and public places"[154] for processions, prayers, and revels. With the relatively recent victories over enemies of Islam--be they Mongols, Franks, or Armenians--Damascus saw a resurgent spirit of holy war that was soon turned inward and transformed into a heightened intolerance for Muslim heresy.[155]

The exact details of the context of suppression of heresy during the period is poorly understood, and this is in part due to the assumptions of scholars that studied it. One of these assumptions led to a tendency to look at the Islamic world through the lens of European institutions that have often been viewed in the context of the state. Eliyahu Ashtor (d. 1984) is the scholar that most closely studied the suppression of heresy in the Mamlūk period. To Ashtor, this endeavor was a form of inquisition carried out by the state in a conscious attempt to avoid theological differences that often gave rise to political and social movements that threatened governments in the Western medieval world.[156] Ashtor was later critiqued for having directly applied Western categories and Western historiography to the Middle East, as well as attributing concerns and intentions to the Mamlūk state that dominated the West. As Chamberlain retorts, there was never

---

[153] Chamberlain, *Knowledge and Social Practice*, 168.
[154] Ira M. Lapidus, *Muslim Cities in the Later Middle Ages* (Cambridge: Cambridge University Press, 1984), 12.
[155] *Ibid.*
[156] Elitayahu Ashtor, "L'inquisition dans l'état mamlouk," *Rivista degli Studi Orientali* 25 (1950): 11-26.

any evidence for "the existence of state or corporate bodies with jurisdiction over heresy."[157] And indeed, when describing the "Mamlūk Inquisition", Ashtor's examples are not representative of an institutional inquisition but of an amalgam of attitudes, reactions, and processes of accusation laid before judges.[158]

While the suppression of heresy cannot be denied as an important aspect of Mamlūk society, the existence of a state-driven tribunal dedicated to an inquisition is a leap. Rather, we should interpret struggle to define correct belief as a form of competition by the urban elites.[159] The *fitnas* that resulted from this find their roots in the instability of the resources of the *amīrs*' households: wealth, power, and prestige were objects of competition as much as the legitimacy of the control over them.[160]

As we will see, many proponents of Prophetic Medicine were members of the Ḥanbalī *madhhab*. The four different schools of jurisprudence in Islamic law were in theory tolerant of each other's beliefs.[161] However, Ḥanbalīs' positions in theological matters often varied a lot from those of other *madhhabs*. Issues like the createdness of the Qur᾿ān, as well as the practice of visiting tombs and the belief in the divine attributes of God, would create a split between the Ḥanbalīs and the other *madhhabs*. This created tensions between them and antagonism toward Ḥanbalīs, whose positions were often more scripturalist than that of their adversaries. In all cases

---

157 Chamberlain, *Knowledge and Social Practice*, 168.
158 Ashtor, "L'inquisition dans l'état mamlouk", 15-20.
159 Chamberlain, *Knowledge and Social Practice*, 168.
160 *Ibid.*, 47.
161 Schacht, *An Introduction to Islamic Law*, 66.

of these *fitnas*, however, state institutions were not implicated: matters of suppression of heresy were not carried out by the ruling elite.[162]

It is thus in part in this context that Prophetic Medicine must be understood. While we must not imagine it as an affirmation that the Prophet's *Sunnā* opposed categorically the kind of medicine that was contemporarily practiced, i.e. Graeco-Islamic medicine, we must understand that it was also developed in the context of a non-institutional reaffirmation of traditionalism by intellectuals and religious elites.

What is meant here by "traditionalism" is the emphasis on the importance of divine revelation and the adherence to the *Sunnā* of the Prophet. Traditionalist elements were present among all the legal schools, but members of the Ḥanbalī legal school formed "the spearhead of the movement", because the teachings of Ibn Ḥanbal had been the most significant expression of the rejection of innovation (*bidʿa*) in favor of scripturalism.[163]

At its core, traditionalism advocated the importance of divine revelation instead of rationalist theology. During the Mamlūk period, the Ashaʿrite school, followers of Abū al-Ḥasan ʿAlī al-Ashʿarī (d. 936), were the main proponents of rational theology. The theology of the traditionalists was instead based on the Qurʾān and on the Sunnā of the Prophet. According to them, explaining issues of dogma could not benefit from rationality because they were matters of faith.[164]

---

[162] For examples of how *fitnas* occurred without the involvement of the ruling elite, see Chamberlain, *Knowledge and Social Practice*, 170-171.
[163] George Makdisi, "Ashʿarī and the Ashʿarites in Islamic Religious History I," *Studia Islamica* 17 (1962): 46.
[164] Montgomery Watt, *Islamic Philosophy and Theology: An Extended Survey* (Edinburgh: Edinburgh University Press, 1985), 64-104.

However, traditionalism did not merely limit its claim to theology and questions of ritual. It also extended its application to issues of moral code, and the sources for the Islamic norms was the corpus of ḥadīths. In this context one of the most notable examples of reformism is the life and the activism of Ḥanbalī scholar Taqī al-Dīn Aḥmad ibn Taymiyya (d. 1328). His teachings were not strictly typical of the Ḥanbalī school of law, but it would be naïve to imagine that his reformism did not influence the course of the development of Prophetic Medicine. For indeed, Ibn Qayyim al-Jawziyya (d. 1348), Shams al-Dīn al-Dhahabī (d. 1350), and Shams al-Dīn Ibn Mufliḥ al-Maqdisī (d. 1362), authors of some of the most comprehensive treatises of Prophetic Medicine, were all associated with the Ḥanbalī school and were students of Ibn Taymiyya.

The traditionalist *ʿulamāʾ* thus wrote religious treatises aimed at refuting the views of the rational theologians, but also wrote treatises that addressed *ḥadīths* and explained them to the public and tracts against *bidʿa* which warned the public about what should be considered impious and exhorted the readers to respect what they considered correct behaviour. Certain works in which some Prophetic Medicine is found include Ibn Qayyīm al-Jawziyya's *Zād al-maʿād fī hadī khayr al-ʿibād Muḥammad*[165] and Ibn Mufliḥ's *al-Ādāb al-sharʿiyya wa-al-minaḥ al-marʿiyya.*[166] The fact that these works of Prophetic Medicine were originally parts of greater works dedicated to publicizing the authors' opinion of correct behaviour is indicative of the possible intent of Prophetic Medicine, and we shall discuss this more fully in the following chapter.

Under the Mamlūks, Damascus had gradually grown into a stronghold of Ḥanbalism, mostly due to two main reasons. First, we should mention the resounding activism of one of the most influential champion of the Ḥanbalī school, Ibn Taymiyya, as well as the work of members

[165] Ibn Qayyim al-Jawziyya, *Zād al-maʿād fī hadī khayr al-ʿibād Muḥammad* (Beirut: Al-Resalah, 1979).
[166] Shams al-Dīn Ibn Mufliḥ al-Maqdisī, *al-Ādāb al-sharʿiyya wa-al-minaḥ al-marʿiyya*, (Egypt: Maṭbaʿat al-Manār, 1930).

of the Banū Munajjā and Banū Qudāma, two of the main dynasties of Ḥanbalī intellectuals and jurists that had settled in Damascus during the Zangid period (1154-1174).[167] Another reason for the growth of the Ḥanbalī school during the first Mamlūk era was the forced immigration from Ḥarrān in Mesopotamia of Ḥanbalī scholars fleeing the yoke of the Mongols.[168] Ḥarrān had been a center of Ḥanbalism, which had its scholars evicted following its conquest by the Mongols.[169]

In Damascus, this period thus brought an increased interest in *ḥadīth* and calls for returning to the Prophet's *Sunnā* (the custom of the Prophet) by certain *Sunnī* scholars like Ibn al-Nafīs (d. 1288), who blamed society's deviations from the *Sunnā* for the Mongol invasion. The punishment from God was delivered through bloodshed because of the sinfulness of the community of the Prophet. Among the sins that this community was made guilty of, Ibn al-Nafīs mentioned the appearance of women in public in the presence of strangers, and drinking of wine, which had become largely used as a remedy.[170] The bloodshed was to come from invading infidels rather than another religious community, "because in this case their success would be regarded as the success of their religion, and that would be contrary to the aim of this punishment."[171] Another example is Ibn al-Ḥājj (d. 1256), who criticized popular Muslim celebrations that he considered innovations from the practice of the Prophet and his close followers.[172]

As we have seen, conservative scholars also attacked the proponents of the "ancient sciences" (*ʿulūm al-awāʾil*), the *falāsifa*. The group of traditionalist *Sunnī* scholars who formulated

[167] Henri Laoust, "Le Hanbalisme sous les Mamlouks Bahrides," *Revue des études islamiques* 28 (1960): 1-54.
[168] Lapidus, *Muslim Cities*, 112.
[169] Henri Laoust, "Le Hanbalisme sous le Califat de Bagdad (241/855 – 656/1258)," *Revue des études islamiques*, 28 (1959): 67-128.
[170] Joseph Schacht and Max Meyerhof, *The Theologus Autodidactus of Ibn al-Nafīs* (Oxford: Clarendon Press, 1968) 96.
[171] *Ibid.*, 97.
[172] Muḥammad ibn Muḥammad ibn al-Ḥājj, *Kitāb al-Madkhal* (Cairo: al-Maṭbaʿa al-Miṣriyya bi-al-Azhar, 1929).

these critiques was described by Dimitri Gutas as made up of conservative Damascene scholars of the Shāfiʿī and Ḥanbalī schools of law whose attitudes were conditioned in part by the Crusades and the Mongol invasion. The effect of these two events was the generation of a less tolerant version of Islam and an exacerbation of an already precarious situation. Attitudes evolved toward aggressive ideological positions against non-Muslims and against heresy, as well as a firmer resurgence of "conservative" traditionalism upheld by Ḥanbalīs like Ibn Taymiyya.[173] These attacks by the *ḥadīth* scholars "who saw themselves as the true guardians of the *sunna*"[174] and "the inheritors of the Prophet's literal words and intention"[175] might have been conditioned by the recent circumstances of the *madrasa*, which gradually incorporated the "ancient sciences."

Mamlūks, Islam, and the Perceptions of Contemporary Historians

At this point it appears necessary to examine more closely the relations between the Mamlūks and religion, and more precisely the relation between the *ʿulamāʾ* and the Mamlūks. These are matters that still have some blind spots, but that have been the objects of studies during the second half of the 20th century. The negative attitude of contemporary Arab chroniclers is well-known, but it may not be accepted unquestionably. Indeed, to some contemporary scholars, the Mamlūks did represent the glory of the true faith, incarnated in the restorers of Islam who saved the caliphate from the heresy of the Mongols and the Franks.[176]

---

173 Dimitri Gutas, *Greek Thought, Arabic Culture: The Graeco-Arabic Translation Movement in Baghdad and Early ʿAbbasid Society (2nd-4th/8th-10th centuries)*, (London: Routledge, 1998), 166-175.
174 Fancy, *Science and Religion in Mamluk Egypt*, 18.
175 Fancy, *Pulmonary Transit and Bodily Resurrection*, 39.
176 Donald Little, "Religion under the Mamluks," *The Muslim World* 73 (1983): 165-167.

Ibn Khaldūn (d. 1406), famous Arab historian and historiographer, offered praise for the Mamlūks, along with their military system based on slavery, saying they had been sent by "Divine Providence" to put an end to the rule of the "Tatar infidels who abolished the Caliphate and wiped out the splendor of the land and replaced the True Faith with Unbelief."[177]

Even after the Mongols converted to Islam, the Mamlūks continued to insist on identifying themselves as the champions of the faith and on identifying the conflicts in which they took part as struggles for the glory of Islam against the enemies of God and his Prophet.[178]

Mamlūks erected monuments that boasted an expressive Islamic character and represented their allegiance to Islam. Stephen Humphreys' study of the architectural landscape of Mamlūk Cairo argues that "under the Mamlūks, the major effort in buildings of prestige was devoted neither to secular structures (e.g., palaces, public baths, *khāns* and caravanserais)" but to institutions dedicated to "communal mystical devotion (*khānaqāhs*, *ribāṭs*, *zāwiyas*), the teaching of law and theology (*madrasas*) and the veneration of the departed, either saints or merely those who had striven to defend and uphold the faith (*turbas*, *mashhads*)."[179]

In the larger scheme of the Islamic world, the Mamlūks also had interests in the sacred places of *Sunnī* Islam, such as Mecca and Medina in the peninsula, and Jerusalem and Hebron in Palestine. As the revivers and protectors of the caliphate, they also assumed the role of guardians of the sites of pilgrimage and sacred shrines.[180] Through delegation to the members of the Qatāda tribe, the Mamlūks were ultimate custodians of the Kaʿba and, as such, they were the ones who

---

[177] Ibn Khaldūn, *Kitāb al-ʿIbar*, trans. by David Ayalon in "Mamlūkiyyāt" *Jerusalem Studies in Arabic and Islam* 2 (1980): 345.
[178] Little, "Religion under the Mamluks," 168.
[179] Stephen Humphreys, "The Expressive Intent of the Mamlūk Architecture of Cairo: A Preliminary Essay," *Studia Islamica* 35 (1972): 69-119.
[180] Little, "Religion under the Mamluks," 170-171.

provided each year the cloth destined to cover the shrine, and their banners were exposed in front of those of other Muslim rulers.[181]

As much as we might imagine that the Mamlūks' religiosity was at the root of these campaigns and patronages, we should not merely take the declared motives at face value. For indeed, important trade routes ran through contested areas of the kingdom, and religious institutions and monuments built by the Mamlūks, as we have explained earlier, often served the political goals of the *amīrs*, either as burial settings or to perpetuate one's name and prestige. Furthermore, patronage of intellectual endeavours helped harmonize their interests with those of influential pious groups and leaders, and protecting pilgrimage sites and providing for the pilgrims themselves secured considerable commercial advantages for the Mamlūks.[182]

In this chapter, we have made some observations concerning the context of 13th-and the 14th-century Egypt and Syria. We have attempted to uncover the diverse ways in which the geo-political circumstances favoured a cultural blossoming in the cities of Cairo and Damascus. These cities had always been important centers of the Middle East, but the Mongol invasions provoked a movement toward these urban areas that assembled people of many cultural backgrounds, religious affiliations, and social status. We have seen how the political system of the Mamlūks encouraged the patronage of intellectual and particularly religious activities. Caught up in the instability of their position in the upper strata of society, the military elite of the Mamlūk society turned to the *waqf*, or religious endowment, in order to secure the integrity of the assets they had amassed. The non-hereditary nature of higher administrative offices and the difficulty of transferring capital, be it social, symbolic or economic, from a patriarch to his descendants

[181] Donald Little, "The History of Arabia during the Baḥrī Mamlūk Period," *Studies in the History of Arabia* 1 (1979): 20.
[182] Little, "Religion Under the Mamlūks," 172.

ultimately brought about a burgeoning of many institutions of knowledge. This situation gave voice to many intellectual debates and certain *Sunnī* scholars criticized contemporary Muslim society and how far it had strayed from the tradition of Muḥammad.

It is against this background that one must see the development of Prophetic Medicine: a background of heightened intellectual and religious activity, but also one of resurgence of traditionalism and skepticism toward the piety of new masters. The Mongols, who represented for many the Divine punishment for the sins of Islamic society, were still a neighboring danger that were a reminder of the imperative to uphold the *Sunnā* of the Prophet. Such exaltation of Syrian Sunnism was primordial in the development of Ḥanbalism under the Mamlūks and it is among this revitalization of traditionalism that Prophetic Medicine was mostly developed.

Chapter 3: The Development of Prophetic Medicine

Now that we have approached some of the main elements that formed the context that was fruitful to the development of Prophetic Medicine, it must be noted that it did not spontaneously sprout out of the 14th century. Indeed, what ended up becoming the interesting result of the combination of religion and science truly finds its roots in the first centuries of Islam. Thus, Prophetic Medicine is above all an evolving category.

In order to make sense of the evolution of Prophetic Medicine, we will present the history of Prophetic Medicine in four stages. However, it must be acknowledged that the development of this genre did not confine itself to this four-stage scheme, and that it was instead a continual process. The boundaries of said stages are thus not impermeable, and also not represented in reality by any event in particular. The model that we shall present here is not a perfect one, and some example of works of Prophetic Medicine do not correspond to the timeline. What we shall attempt to present here is a heuristic device meant to familiarize ourselves with a development that spanned over more than eight centuries. These stages are based on observable changes in the content and the form of the works: early examples of the genre will exhibit almost no references to Greek medicine and medical theories, while later examples will gradually include more Graeco-Islamic medical theory that was simultaneously growing in influence.

What we shall attempt to demonstrate here is that the nature of Prophetic Medicine gradually evolved to engage more directly with contemporary medical theory and practice. From uncommented collections of Prophetic reports by authors only marginally interested in medical matters, Prophetic Medicine becomes, around the 13th and 14th centuries, a distinct genre of medico-religious literature that offers a complete system. As we will see, Prophetic Medicine, even in its most "mature" form, did not attempt to replace the medicine of "the physicians", but to modify, to adjust it, so that it would respect Islamic doctrine as defined in the Qurʾān and in the words of the Prophet.

The First Stage (8th-9th c.)

The first stage of the development of the genre of Prophetic Medicine is what we could describe as a "proto-" Prophetic Medicine. At this stage, it might still be too early to carry the name because it does not share many of the characteristics of the "end-product" of our timeline, but it must be recognized as its precursor. The 8th-9th centuries are often referred to as the formative period of Islamic law, and during this period, the Prophet's sayings came to be accepted as sources of law in addition to the Qurʾān. The usage of *ḥadīths* was not limited to deriving law, but also contributed in providing a prescriptive and normative example of everyday life for Muslims.

As we have seen in the previous chapter, the importance of *ḥadīths* was invaluable, along with the Qurʾān, in the process of determining matters of dogma, ritual and daily practice. Thus, by the 8th century, there were two main positions concerning the interpretation of Islam, the source of which were the Qurʾān and the Prophet, which itself was carried by the Companions, i.e. the Muslims that had seen the Prophet while he was alive.

On the one hand, when a new situation arrived, or when the sources were not clear, certain scholars like Abū Ḥanīfa (d. 772) relied on their own interpretations of these sources. These were known as the *ahl al-raʾy* ("Partisans of Legal Reasoning").

On the other hand, certain scholars like Aḥmad ibn Ḥanbal (d. 855), preferred to rely on "the opinions of the earliest generations of Muslims and more dubious reports from the Prophet rather than speculate in a realm they felt was the exclusive purview of God and His Prophet."[183] These scholars were known as *ahl al-ḥadīth* ("Partisans of Ḥadīth"). "For them," explains Jonathan Brown, "the Muslim confrontation with the cosmopolitan atmosphere of the Near East threatened the unadulterated purity of Islam."[184]

The first compilations of *ḥadīths* took the form of *saḥīfas*, small notebooks that presented a skeleton of a report from the Prophet. In the context of a tradition focused on orality, these were designed so they would spark the memory of the one reading it to his audience. The most prolific collector of the sort was Abū Hurayra (d. 678), with around 5,300 *ḥadīths*.[185] The *Muwaṭṭa'* of Mālik ibn Anas (d. 796) is an example of the first topically organized works of *ḥadīths* compilation. These were called *muṣannafs*, and included Prophetic *ḥadīths*, Companions' opinions, practice of contemporary scholars, and opinions of the author.[186] The *musnad* collections emerged in the late 8th and early 9th centuries, and shifted the focus from the topic to the authenticity, thus organizing the reports according to their *isnād*, their chain of transmission.[187] The two genres were combined by esteemed members of the *ahl al-ḥadīth* in the form of *sunan* / *saḥīḥ* books, which were collections that were organized topically and provided full *isnāds*.[188]

Ḥadīths were thus collected in very extensive books, and in the *Saḥīḥ* of al-Bukhārī, the ones that pertained to health, medicine, sickness, and patients were put together in separate

---

183 Jonathan Brown, *Ḥadīth: Muḥammad's Legacy in the Medieval and Modern World* (London: Oneworld, 2014), 17.
184 *Ibid.*
185 *Ibid.*, 18-24.
186 *Ibid.*, 25-27.
187 *Ibid.*, 28-30.
188 *Ibid.*, 31-34.

chapters. For example, the collection of al-Bukhārī known as *al-Ṣaḥīḥ al-Bukhārī* contained a chapter titled *Kitāb al-Marḍā* ("The Book of the Sick") and one titled *Kitāb al-Ṭibb* ("The Book of Medicine").[189] Another instance of such chapters can be found in *Sunan ibn Māja*, titled *Kitāb al-Marḍā*.[190]

The *ḥadīth* content of these chapters is relatively not wide ranging, and consists of many versions of the same Prophetic injunctions. In order to grasp the nature of their medical content, we provide a brief overview of medicine as included in the collections of the *sunān/saḥīḥ* type, and take as an example the *Saḥīḥ al-Bukhārī*. The many books of the collection of al-Bukhārī present various subjects of *fiqh* ("jurisprudence"), but is also includes many other matters such as the Creation, paradise and hell, different prophets, details on Muḥammad and on Qur'ān commentary, etc.

The chapters that are of interest to us are chapters 70 and 71, respectively titled *Kitāb al-Marḍā* (*Book of the Sick*) and *Kitāb al-Ṭibb* (*Book of Medicine*). The first one contains 22 *abwāb* ("chapters", sing. *bāb*), while the second contains 58 *abwāb*. Each *bāb* regroups the *ḥadīths* that pertain to the matter announced in its title, which itself indicates "the legal implication or ruling the reader should derive from the subsequent *ḥadīths*."[191] Al-Bukhārī provides between one and six *ḥadīths* per bāb as well as the *isnād* for each of them, and many *ḥadīths* are used in more than one *bāb*.[192]

---

[189] Muḥammad ibn Ismā'īl al-Bukhārī, *The Translation of the Meanings of Ṣaḥīḥ al-Bukhārī: Arabic-English*, trans. Muhammad Muhsin Khan, (Chicago: Kazi Publications, 1979), 371-453.
[190] Ibn Māja, *Sunan Ibn Māja* (Beirut: Dar al-Kutub al-'Ilmiyyah, 1987), 2:1137-1175.
[191] Jonathan Brown, *The Canonization of al-Bukhārī and Muslim: The Formation and Function of the Sunnī Ḥadīth Canon* (Leiden: Brill, 2007), 69.
[192] Al-Bukhārī, *The Translation of the Meanings*, 371-453.

There appeared to be no precise order in the arrangement of the topics that are covered. However, it is worthwhile to point out that there are two general, sometimes overlapping, types of *ḥadīths* in the two books that are of interest to us. The first type, and the most common in the chapters that we examine, corresponds to *ḥadīths* concerned with practice, in the sense that they oblige, specify, or recommend an action. For example, much of the *Book of the Sick* revolves around the obligation of Muslims to visit the sick.[193] In fact, 11 out of the 22 *abwāb* of this book refer to this duty and set different parameters for it[194], approaching matters like visiting an unconscious patient,[195] a sick child,[196] a sick Bedouin,[197] or a sick pagan,[198] performing ablution in the stead of a sick person,[199] how a visitor should act[200] and what he should say and what a patient should answer,[201] etc.

In the *Book of Medicine*, the clear majority of the quoted material refers to different practices of medicine, drugs, and treatments. The repetition of variations of the *ḥadīth* stating that there is cure in three things, namely honey, cupping and cautery, but that the Prophet forbids cautery, is noteworthy.[202] Many *ḥadīths* therein discuss the use of drugs, like the milk of camels[203] and she-asses,[204] the urine of camels,[205] black cumin,[206] *talbīna* (a compound of milk, honey and

---

[193] *Ibid.*, 375 (*ḥadīths* no. 552, 554)
[194] *Ibid.*, 371-394.
[195] *Ibid.*, 376 (554).
[196] *Ibid.*, 378 (559).
[197] *Ibid.*, 379 (570).
[198] *Ibid.*, 380 (561).
[199] *Ibid.*, 393 (580).
[200] *Ibid.*, 381-383 (562-564).
[201] *Ibid.*, 383-393 (565, 566, 579).
[202] *Ibid.*, 396 (585-588, 603, 605, 606).
[203] *Ibid.*, 398 (589).
[204] *Ibid.*, 451-452 (672).
[205] *Ibid.*, 399 (590).
[206] *Ibid.*, 399-400 (591-592).

flour),[207] *su'ūt* (medicine sniffed by nose),[208] *qusṭ* (a type of incense),[209] antimony,[210] truffles,[211] *ladūd* (medicine inserted in the side of the mouth),[212] ashes of palm-tree leaves[213] and *'ajwa* dates.[214] Some *ḥadīths* present details about treatment by cupping[215] or with *ruqā* (recitation of Divine verses).[216] Some reports present things that a Muslim should not do, and are against soothsaying[217] or magic.[218]

Ḥadīths of the second type state a belief, a certain conceptualization, or an epistemological guidance, and there are considerably less reports of this type. In the *Book of Patients* is stated the belief that sickness is expiation for sins and that "whoever works evil will have the recompense thereof."[219] The belief that sickness is an ordeal from God and that, while relatively uncomfortable, it is ultimately a good thing and a sign of piety, is the subject of many variations.[220]

The *Book of Medicine* presents a more varied set of beliefs that are mandatory for Muslims. First, the statement that there is no *'adwā* ("contagion") takes the front.[221] The other statements of beliefs that are included in this work concerning medicine are the belief that God has not created a disease without creating its treatment as well,[222] that fever is from the heat of Hell,[223] that "the

---

207 *Ibid.*, 401 (593-594).
208 *Ibid.*, 401-402 (595).
209 *Ibid.*, 402 (596).
210 *Ibid.*, 408 (607).
211 *Ibid.*, 409 (608).
212 *Ibid.*, 409-410 (610-611).
213 *Ibid.*, 415-416 (618).
214 *Ibid.*, 446-451 (663-664, 671).
215 *Ibid.*, 402-405 (597-603).
216 *Ibid.*, 423-435 (631-635, 637-648)
217 *Ibid.*, 437-440 (654-657).
218 *Ibid.*, 440-446 (658-664).
219 *Ibid.*, 371.
220 *Ibid.*, 371-392 (544-551, 555-557, 575-578).
221 *Ibid.*, 413-447 (615, 665-668).
222 *Ibid.*, 395 (582).
223 *Ibid.*, 416-417 (619-622).

effect of an evil eye is a fact,"[224] that there is no *ṭiyara* (i.e. the drawing of evil omen from birds, etc.)[225]

Many of the statements that introduce each *bāb* appear to be quite vague, such as the one stating that the evil eye is real, etc. Consequently, many contradictions are left for the jurists to interpret, such as the statement that there is no such thing as contagion, faced with the report that the Prophet told his followers not to put a patient with healthy person,[226] etc.

Through this, we can glimpse at the position that al-Bukhārī seems to take when collecting *ḥadīths*: that of a somewhat neutral agent. Indeed, it was never determined whether he had taken a position with one legal school or another, but each school, even the Ḥanafīs who declined the use of *ḥadīths*, came to claim him as one of their own.[227] We thus come to a conclusion that supports that of J. Robson that al-Bukhārī was an independent author and never consistently abided by the principles of one single *madhhab*.[228] Scott C. Lucas' analysis of al-Bukhārī's legal theory reveals that the 9th century compilator was not affiliated with one of the major *sunnī* legal schools. To Lucas, al-Bukhārī's work stood out for its absolute commitment to the highest quality *ḥadīths* and its disapproving stance on *qiyās* ("analogical reasoning").[229] As such, it can be seen as a modest precursor to "classical Salafi Islam" normally dated back only to Ibn Taymiyya and Ibn Qayyim al-Jawziyya.[230]

---

[224] *Ibid.*, 426-427 (636).
[225] *Ibid.*, 435-436 (649-651).
[226] *Ibid.*, 447 (665).
[227] Brown, *Canonization*, 71.
[228] J. Robson, "al-Bukhārī, Muḥammad b. Ismā'īl," in *Encyclopedia of Islam, 2nd edition*, edited by P. Bearman, Th. Bianquis, C.E. Bosworth, E. van Donzel and W.P. Heinrichs (Leiden: Brill, 2012), accessed April 12th, 2017, http://dx.doi.org/10.1163/1573-3912_islam_SIM_1510.
[229] Scott Lucas, "The Legal Principles of Muhammad B. Ismā'īl al-Bukhārī and their Relationship to Classical Salafi Islam," *Islamic Law and Society* 13 (2006): 291-297.
[230] *Ibid.*, 290.

However, this is not to say that he did not provide his opinion on the way the *sunna* (the tradition of the Prophet, his words and actions, and that which had been said and done in his presence) should be interpreted, for, as we have seen, almost every *ḥadīth* was completed by his suggestion of what to derive from it. As explained by Lucas, al-Bukhārī's *Ṣaḥīḥ* was a practical articulation of his legal theory, and thus constituted "[one] of the only books of substantive law in the Islamic tradition constructed exclusively upon the Qur'ān and sound prophetic *ḥadīths*."[231]

This is significant because it hints at the motives of such endeavors of collecting reports about the Prophet and the Companions. This was not a matter of taking part in the debates over the theological interpretation and the epistemological role of the *sunna*, but rather more of an attempt to present in a concise manner what is expected of every Muslim. And indeed, this brief analysis highlighted the relative importance of orthopraxy in sickness and treatment: while the two books do convey some information about what is "correct" belief concerning the conceptualization of sickness, health, and cure, the insistence truly is on practice.

Throughout these two books of the collection, one of the recurrent themes is that sickness, cure and health are somewhat divine. God is responsible for all three states, and between naturalistic methods of healing and super-naturalistic ones like magic, we see that it is through his creation that God provides healing. It is therefore possible to suppose that the Prophetic actions and utterances did not necessarily came into direct conflict with the medical theory of the Greeks, which emphasized natural causality, environment, habits, etc. This divine nature of the states of health and sickness and of the process of healing may also point to one of the reasons that led to

[231] *Ibid.*, 321.

the development of Prophetic Medicine. Health and sickness are part of the realm of the divine, and as such, should not escape the prescriptions of revelation.

On the other hand, at a first glance, we can imagine that *ḥadīth* literature from the 9th century was far from enough to guide the believers in their experience of disease and cure, and this might have had an impact on the how ready Muslims were to adopt and adapt the Greek medical heritage. This will become interesting when we shall present the overview of the second stage in the development of Prophetic Medicine. During this stage, we begin to see an increasing amount of medical theory making its way into collections of medical *ḥadīths*. This is significant with regard to our assessment of the first stage for two reasons. Firstly, when looking at the medical content of *ḥadīths* collections of the 8th and 9th centuries, one could find that a lot is missing. Merely a dozen substances are proposed as medicaments for an also quite limited amount of illnesses and conditions treated. Secondly and ultimately, not much is mentioned concerning the conceptualization of sickness, medicine, and health.

These works including chapters dedicated to the medical sayings of the Prophet support the idea that what existed at that point must be set as a background to the later development of Prophetic Medicine, but it would be relatively difficult to make them fit into the parameters of Prophetic Medicine, which will truly become clear as we make our way through its history. In other words, this stage must be understood as an ancestor of Prophetic Medicine and can be explained by a simple concern of the early *ḥadīths* collectors to sort the sayings thematically. At this point, there is no medical theory included with the *ḥadīths*. This, along with the rarity of interpretations of the sayings, suggest that during this period, what we have in terms of the convergence of *ḥadīths* and medicine is far from what we could call a medical system or a circumscribed genre of literature.

The collections of medical *ḥadīths* included in the greater scope of the *saḥīḥs* collections of 9th century scholars did not carry the name of *ṭibb al-nabawī* ("medicine of the Prophet"). However, according to Perho, the first book to ever be titled *Kitāb al-ṭibb al-nabawī* was written by ʿAbd al-Malik ibn Ḥabīb al-Sulamī al-Qurṭubī (d. 853). Al-Qurṭubī was a philologist, poet and historian from Andalusia.[232] His book has unfortunately not survived and its content is not known.[233] However, another work titled *Kitāb ṭibb al-nabawī ʿalā raʾy ahl al-bayt* ("Prophetic Medicine According to the Opinion of the House of the Prophet") might have been written even earlier by Abū Mūsā Jābir ibn Ḥayyān who died in 815.[234] Born in Ṭūs in Iran, Jābir ibn Ḥayyān was a renowned polymath and alchemist and worked, among other things, as a physician and a pharmacist. The authorship of many of his works has however been disputed since the 10th century.[235] As Paul Kraus has demonstrated, many of the works ascribed to him might have not been his.[236]

The Second Stage (10th-12th c.)

The second stage of the development of Prophetic Medicine occurred during the 10th, 11th and 12th centuries. During this phase, the works that we can identify as belonging to the larger definition of Prophetic Medicine seem to start being organized differently. The influence of the

---

232 Carl Brockelmann, *Geschichte der Arabischen Litteratur*, 2nd edition (Leiden: Brill, 1945), 1:156. [Hereafter abbreviated *GAL*]

233 Ömer Recep, *Tibb an-Nabī: die Prophetenmedizin bei Ibn as-Sunnī und Abū Nuʿaim unter besonderer Ber□cksichtigung der Kapitel □ber den Kopfschmerz, die Augen-, Nasen-, Zahnkrankheiten und die H□morrhoiden* (Marburg/Lahn: E. Symon, 1969), 4.

234 Paul Kraus, *Jābir ibn Hayyān, contribution à l'histoire des idées scientifiques dans l'Islam: Jābir et la science grecque* (Paris: Belles Lettres, 1986), 1:95.

235 Tod Brabner, "Jabir ibn Ḥayyān (Geber)," in *Medieval science, Technology, and Medicine: An Encyclopedia*, edited by Thomas F. Glick, Steven John Livesey and Faith Wallis, (New York: Routledge, 2005), 279-281.

236 Kraus, *Jābir ibn Hayyān*, XLVI-XLVIII.

growth of the main genre of medicine accepted in the Islamic world, i.e. Graeco-Islamic medicine, starts to be felt in the books that regroup the opinions of the Prophet concerning medical matters and health.

Among the works that were produced during this phase, the *Geschichte des arabischen Schrifttums* of Fuat Sezgin mentions that of Aḥmad ibn Muḥammad al-Dinawarī, also known as Ibn al-Sunnī (d. 974), titled *Ṭibb al-nabī.*[237] This might currently be the oldest surviving book of Prophetic Medicine.[238] However, Maḥmūd Nāẓim al-Nasīmī, author of an extent study on Prophetic Medicine, claims that the book itself has not survived.[239] Ömer Recep, claims that Ibn al-Sunnī wrote an abridged version of his own work and it is that which survived and was mistaken for the original.[240]

Among the early texts, al-Nasīmī also mentions the *Ṭibb al-nabī* of Abū al-ʿAbbās Jaʿfar ibn Muḥammad al-Mustaghfirī al-Nasafī (d. 1041), Hanafī jurist and preacher.[241] The *Ṭibb al-nabī* of Abū Nuʿaym al-Iṣfahānī (d. 1038) is also of this period.[242] Al-Iṣfahānī was a Shāfiʿī scholar and historian and was considered among the best *ḥadīth* authorities of his time, but it is mostly due to his *Ḥilyat al-awliyāʾ wa-ṭabaqāt al-aṣfiyāʾ* that he acquired an influential posthumous reputation. The *Ḥilyat* was "a vast compilation of prophetic utterances and traditions attributed to individuals from the earliest days of Islam onwards, who, according to [al-Iṣfahānī], were regarded as ascetics

---

237 Fuat Sezgin, *Geschichte des arabischen Schrifttums* (Leiden: Brill, 1967), 1:198.
238 Perho, *The Prophet's Medicine*, 54.
239 Maḥmūd Nāẓim al-Nasīmī, *al-Ṭibb al-nabawī wa-ʿIlm al-ḥadīth*, (Beirut: Mūʾassasat al-Risālah, 1987), 30.
240 Recep, *Tibb an-Nabī*, 4-5.
241 al-Nasīmī, *al-Ṭibb al-nabawī*, 1:46; Carl Brockelmann, *Geschichte der arabischen Litteratur Supplementbänden*, (Leiden: Brill, 1937-1942), 1:617. [Hereafter abbreviated *GALS*]
242 *GAL*, 1:362; *GALS*, 1:616.

and mystics."[243] His work on the medicine of the Prophet is among his smaller but numerous works connected to his expertise as a traditionist.[244]

The significance of al-Iṣfahānī's *Ṭibb al-nabī* is, among other things, its extent. Boasting 838 *ḥadīths*, it was the largest compilation of medical *ḥadīths* yet. This number is however explained by the fact that he quoted many variations of the same *ḥadīths*. For example, he gives as many as 26 variations of the saying that states that "for every illness there is a cure,"[245] and certain headings contain as many as 40 *ḥadīths*, compared to a maximum of three per heading in Ibn al-Sunnī's work.[246] The extent of al-Iṣfahānī's book has contributed to make it a prime source for later authors.[247]

The interesting evolution that is realized in this phase pertains to the organization of the *ḥadīths* that are reported. Indeed, in the arrangement of their subject matter, they followed the organization of the contemporary medical books: first presenting chapters on illnesses of the head and then working their way down to the illnesses of the feet.[248]

To explain this evolution, Perho proposes that there must have been a concern for creating something that would make the books of Prophetic Medicine appealing to physicians that were not necessarily interested in *ḥadīths* collections. Making their works available to a larger public would have been profitable as well as promoting a medical practice that would be more in line with

[243] Jacqueline Chabbi, "Abū Nuʿaym al-Iṣfahānī," in *Encyclopaedia of Islam*, 3rd edition, edited by Kate Fleet, Gudrun Krämer, Denis Matringe, John Nawas, Everett Rowson. (Leiden: Brill, 2011), accessed on April 8th, 2017, http://dx.doi.org/10.1163/1573-3912_ei3_COM_23648.
[244] *Ibid.*
[245] Recep, *Tibb an-Nabī*, 2-11 [of the Arabic text].
[246] *Ibid.*, 20.
[247] Perho, *The Prophet's Medicine*, 54.
[248] al-Nasīmī, *al-Ṭibb al-nabawī*, 1:43.

Muslim concerns.[249] From that moment on, Prophetic Medicine was not only the concern of *ḥadīths* scholars and Muslim jurists, but also that of physicians.

Another conclusion that can be drawn from a look into these works is that the authors were indeed no physicians: their main interest was still the compilation and the presentation of *ḥadīths* themselves. The compiling of the reports of the Prophet's and his companions' utterances had for a long time been an important activity of Muslim scholars. The compilation of *ḥadīths* emerged as a "practical solution to the needs of the Muslim community"[250] in terms of the elaboration of Islamic law and dogma and as "a form of connection to the Prophet's charismatic legacy."[251] As such, a scholar that could boast authorship of such a work enjoyed a special recognition in the eyes of his peers and those of the general public. Since the nature of religious authority in Islam is such that it emanates from God through his Prophet, claiming a connection to the latter as an inheritor of his tradition could bestow authority with regards to correct belief and behaviour. Eerik Dickinson, speaking of the role of the *isnād* in the thought of Ibn Ṣalāḥ al-Shahrazūrī (d. 1245) and later *ḥadīth* scholars, explains that the "proximity to the Prophet had special significance because it was seen as indicative of spiritual superiority."[252]

No analysis of the medical issues related to the quoted reports is presented in these books. There is yet no attempt to present the scriptural prescriptions in the form of a coherent and complete system, and the reports are not accompanied by any medical theory. Thus, one may not

---

249 Perho, *The Prophet's Medicine*, 56.
250 Brown, *Ḥadīth*, 15.
251 *Ibid*.
252 Eerik Dickinson, "Ibn al-Ṣalāḥ al-Shahrazūrī and the Isnād," *Journal of the American Oriental Society* 122, no. 3 (2002): 505.

qualify these as medical texts, but rather as *hadīths* collection that are merely specialized in medical topics.

The Third Stage (12th-13th c.)

The third phase of the development of Prophetic Medicine begins toward the end of the 12th century. To an extent, this is the period during which the genre of Prophetic medicine matures and truly starts to become itself in a general sense: during this phase, the texts tend to present increasingly common characteristics with the most known works of Prophetic Medicine that appear in the 14th century, during the ultimate phase of development. In the third and fourth stages, Prophetic Medicine slowly evolves into a proper genre of medical literature. It must not be misunderstood that what we would refer to as the stages of this development are actually processes in themselves. During this third stage of the process, authors of Prophetic Medicine gradually start to include Graeco-Islamic medical theory in their *ḥadīth* collections.

The first example of this development is the *Kitāb luqaṭ al-manāfiʿ fī al-ṭibb* of ʿAbd al-Raḥmān ibn al-Jawzī (d. 1200).[253] In this example, we find slightly fewer reports from the Prophet than in the works of his predecessors, and their content is not analysed or interpreted medically. However, illnesses and cures are presented in the same order as they are in contemporary medical books: from head to toe, and the work does present an explanation of Graeco-Islamic medical theory.[254]

253 *GAL*, 1:505; *GALS*, 1:920.
254 Perho, *The Prophet's Medicine*, 55.

As mentioned above, our separation of the phases is not clean cut and absolute. Even though Ibn al-Jawzī's *Luqaṭ* was probably the first one to present the characteristics of the later evolution of the genre, at this early moment of the third stage, there are still works being written that must be qualified as simple *ḥadīth* collections without commentary. Ibn al-Jawzī's pupil, Ḍiyā' al-Dīn Muḥammad ibn ʿAbd al-Wāḥid ibn Aḥmad al-Maqdisī al-Ḥanbalī (d. 1245), was the author of a very short treatise titled *al-Ṭibb al-nabawī*, which was too short to include any medical theory or interpretation of *ḥadīths*.[255]

Also in this category are the works of Muwaffaq al-Dīn ʿAbd al-Laṭīf al-Baghdādī (d. 1231) and that of Shams al Dīn Muḥammad ibn Abī al-Fatḥ al-Baʿlī (d. 1309). The compilation of al-Baghdādī was put together by one of his students, Muḥammad ibn Yūsuf al-Birzālī (d. 1239), who had travelled to Damascus in order to further his studies of *ḥadīths* with al-Baghdādī, and was titled *al-Arbaʿīn al-ṭibbiyya al-mustakhraja min sunan Ibn Māja wa sharḥuhā li-al-ʿallāma al-ṭabīb ʿAbd al-Laṭīf al-Baghdādī ʿamala tilmīdhuhu al-shaykh Muḥammad ibn Yūsuf al-Birzālī* ("Forty Medical Traditions Taken from the Sunan of Ibn Māja and their Commentary by the Doctor ʿAbd al-Laṭīf al-Baghdādī, Prepared by his Student Muḥammad ibn Yūsuf al-Birzālī"). This work did include commentaries of the *ḥadīths* cited, but did not seem to aspire to comprehensiveness and exhaustiveness in any way: it is still merely a *ḥadīth* collection, not an attempt at creating a medical system.[256] Instead, Perho suggests that, since al-Birzālī was never known as a physician but rather as a *ḥadīth* scholar, his motive "was to gain religious merit and not to create a new form of medicine."[257]

---

[255] *Ibid*., 56.
[256] al-Nasīmī, *al-Ṭibb al-nabawī*, 1:47-54.
[257] Perho, *The Prophet's* Medicine, 56.

The work of al-Baʿlī, titled *al-Ṭibb al-nabawī*, contains forty *ḥadīths* of a medical nature with short commentaries without any medical theory. Along with the previously cited work of al-Birzālī based on the teachings of al-Baghdādī, these works of Prophetic Medicine belong to a very specific genre of *ḥadīth* literature named *Arbaʿīn* ("forty") literature. The works of this type share the characteristic that they contain a selection of forty *ḥadīths*. It has been suggested that the reasons for this limitation that the compilers of this genre imposed on their work stemmed from the cultural significance of the number forty in different Aryan, Semitic and Turanian traditions, and its occurrences in the Qurʾān and the *sunna* of the Prophet. Among others, the number forty was thought to convey the idea of completeness.[258]

In the case of *ḥadīths* transmission, however, the importance of the number forty seems to have had a more direct and applied significance. As stated in many of the works of this type, the reason for the limitation of their compilations was a particular report from the Prophet exhorting Muslims to memorize and propagate forty *ḥadīths*: "Any one who preserves for my community forty traditions relating to religious matters will be raised by Allāh as a *faqīh* ("jurist"). I shall be a witness for him and intercede on his behalf on the day of resurrection."[259] These compilations of forty *ḥadīths* were thus either general or focused on a specific subject.[260] In the latter case, when the subject was medicine, they did not contain any medical theory or medical explanation of the reports; as such, we must identify them as specialized compilations of traditions rather than medical treatises.

---

258 Khalid Alavi, "The Concept of Arbaʿīn and its Basis in the Islamic Tradition," *Islamic Studies* 22, no. 3 (1983), 71-75.
259 Alavi, "The Concept of Arbaʿīn", 75-76.
260 *Ibid.*, 71.

Another student of al-Baghdādī participated in the genre. Aḥmad ibn Yūsuf al-Tifāshī (d. 1253) is the author of *al-Shifā' fī al-ṭibb al-musnad 'an al-sayyid al-muṣṭafā* ("Cure in the Medicine Transmitted from the Prophet"), which was essentially an abridged version of the *Ṭibb al-nabawī* of al-Iṣfahānī. This further attests to the importance and the reach of al-Iṣfahānī and allows us to point out an aspect of the evolution. While al-Tifāshī did not include any medical theory or comments on the reports, the main difference between his and al-Iṣfahānī's compilation is that he left out the chains of transmission and did not repeat the same traditions under various subdivisions.[261] Thus, this may suggest that we are witnessing a shift in the nature of the interest for medical *ḥadīths*.

'Alī ibn 'Abd al-Karīm ibn Tarkhān ibn Taqī al-Ḥamawī, commonly known as 'Alā' al-Dīn al-Kaḥḥāl ibn Ṭarkhān (d. 1320), was a practising doctor who lived in Ṣafad in Palestine.[262] His work of Prophetic Medicine is titled *al-Aḥkām al-nabawiyya fī al-ṣinā' al-ṭibbiyya* ("The Prophet's Decisions in the Medical Art").[263] This book is also part of the *Arba'īn* literature, as it contains exactly forty reports and justifies this in its introduction with the words of the Prophet enjoining the believers to remember forty traditions. In addition to the forty traditions, the book also lists 83 drugs and foodstuffs that were mentioned or used by the Prophet. Ibn Ṭarkhān's work is also distinguished by the extent of its sources, which include extracts of a medical nature from the six standard *ḥadīth* collections (the *Ṣaḥīḥs* of al-Bukhārī and Muslim, the *Sunans* of Abū Dā'ūd, Ibn Māja, al-Tirmidhī and al-Nisā'ī), Mālik's *al-Muwaṭṭa'* and earlier works of Prophetic Medicine like that of Ibn al-Sunnī, al-Iṣfahānī and al-Baghdādī. Along with these *ḥadīth* sources,

---

261 Perho, *The Prophet's Medicine*, 56- 57.
262 *Ibid.*, 57.
263 Recep, *Tibb an-Nabī*, 13.

he also quoted medical authorities like Ibn Sīnā and al-Rāzī in his commentaries.[264] This is a significant evolution that points to the gradual merging of the two medical traditions – medicine in *ḥadīths* and Graeco-Islamic medicine – and to the possible compatibility between them.

Authors of Prophetic Medicine were thus not always *ḥadīth* scholars writing about medicine. Sometimes, and particularly in the later period, they were practicing physicians writing about *ḥadīths*, as was the case with al-Baghdadi and Ibn Ṭarkhān. This further supports the suggestion made by revisionist historians, who insist that Prophetic Medicine was not fundamentally at odds with Graeco-Islamic medicine.

The Fourth Stage (13th-14th c.)

The last phase of the development brings forth, in the 13th-14th centuries, the most extensive works of the genre, and represent the elements that would define Prophetic Medicine. Among these works, we notably find the following: the *al-Ṭibb al-nabawī* of Shams al-Dīn al-Dhahabī (d. 1348)[265], a work of the same title by Ibn Qayyim al-Jawziyya (d. 1350), and the *al-Ādāb al-shar'iyya wa-al-minaḥ al-mar'iyya* of Muḥammad ibn Mufliḥ al-Maqdisī (d. 1362). It is with these works, and especially that of Ibn Qayyim al-Jawziyya, as we will see in the next section of this chapter, that we could say that Prophetic Medicine becomes a medical system of its own. One

[264] Perho, *The Prophet's Medicine*, 57.
[265] Elgood, *Tibb ul-Nabbi or Medicine of the Prophet*. The work translated by Cyril Elgood and attributed al-Suyūṭī has in fact been misidentified. According to Emilie Savage-Smith, F. Klein-Franke and Ming Zhu, this work of Prophetic Medicine was in fact that of Shams al-Dīn al-Dhahabī (d. 1348). Emilie Savage-Smith, Klein-Franke, F. and Zhu, Ming, "Ṭibb," in *Encyclopaedia of Islam*, 2nd edition, edited by P. Bearman, Th. Bianquis, C.E. Bosworth, E. van Donzel, W.P. Heinrichs (Leiden: Brill, 2012), accessed May 2nd, 2017, http://dx.doi.org/10.1163/1573-3912_islam_COM_1216. Furthermore, the author of the translated work mentions having been directly in the presence of more than one Damascene scholars that had all died before al-Suyūṭī's birth in 1445, Elgood, 129. For an in-depth analysis of the authorship of the work of which Cyril Elgood's work is a translation, see Perho, *The Prophet's Medicine*, 36-40.

could even argue for the placement of Ibn Qayyim al-Jawziyya's treatise in its own separate category because of the particular critical engagement that it represented.

The content of the works in these treatises further merged Prophetic tradition with medical theory and practice from the Galenic tradition that had been taken up and assimilated in the Islamic world. The first example of this development is the *al-Ṭibb al-nabawī* of al-Dhahabī, which is similar to the *Luqaṭ* of Ibn al-Jawzī in that it is "a fairly comprehensive medical handbook."[266] However, it differs from its precursor because it refers to the Prophet far more often. Al-Dhahabī, contrary to Ibn al-Jawzī, could avail himself of the works of the physicians al-Baghdādī and Ibn Ṭarkhān. While Ibn al-Jawzī limits the Prophet's authority to religious cures, such as prayer, al-Dhahabī further merges the traditions to the purely medical issues.[267]

The *al-Ṭibb al-nabawī* of al-Dhahabī was divided into three parts. The first part presented theoretical issues from Greek medical theory, such as the elements (*arkān*) and their qualities (fire is hot and dry, air is hot and wet, water is cold and wet, and earth is cold and dry) (*banāt al-arkān*), the temperaments (evenly balanced; majoritarily hot, cold, damp or dry; mixed) (*mizāj*) and the humors (blood, phlegm, yellow bile and black bile). With this system are presented reports from the Prophet and the Companions attesting to the perfect balance of the temperaments of the Prophet. Indeed, al-Dhahabī stated that Muḥammad was the most evenly balanced because his character was the most balanced, and "the more perfectly balanced is the temperament of the body, the better is the nature of the character."[268]

---

266 Perho, *The Prophet's Medicine*, 58.
267 *Ibid.*
268 Elgood, *Tibb ul-Nabbi*, 49.

Other common principles of Greek medical theory are presented by the authors of this phase, such as the Natural, Vital and Psychic faculties and the causes of disease (air, food and drink, bodily movement and reset, emotional movement and rest, waking and sleeping, and excretion and retention), which are mentioned and agreed upon, but not thoroughly discussed. In most cases, many *ḥadīths* are cited to support the principles presented.[269]

The second part of al-Dhahabī's work is dedicated to principles of treatments. In this section, he first presents general guidelines for the administration of medicaments and then presents an alphabetical list of drugs and foodstuffs accompanied with their humoral properties and their use for treating certain illnesses. Many mentioned substances are supported by reports from the Companions of the Prophet, stating how they witnessed their use by the Prophet. Consider this example of the heart of the Palm Tree (*jummār*):

> "Jummār: The heart of the Date Palm is white, cold & wet. It is good for diarrhoea and is slow to be digested.
>
> According to Ibn ʿUmr there was brought to the Prophet the heart of the palm. He said: Among trees there is one tree blessed like the blessedness of the True Believers. By this he meant the Palm Tree. This tradition is given by al-Bukhārī and Muslim."[270]

In this excerpt, a physical description is given, followed by the humoral characteristics of the substance. Then, al-Dhahabī mentions what medical use it is known to have, and relates a tradition found in al-Bukhārī and Muslim that attest to the approval of the Prophet. These are the

---

[269] *Ibid.*, 51-52.
[270] *Ibid.*, 77.

most common elements of the medical compendia of Prophetic Medicine, but are not always present for each substance. For example, "Balūṭ: The acorn is cold & dry. It helps a bedwetter."[271] This example states the properties and the use, but does not present the Prophet's opinion of it. Other examples do not contain the opinion of the Prophet, but rather that of famous Greek doctors:

> "Jūz: The walnut is hot & dry. It causes headaches. It is difficult to digest and is bad for the stomach. The fresh walnut is better than the dried. A confection of walnuts & honey is good for pains in the throat.
>
> Said Avicenna: To eat figs, walnuts, and rue is a remedy for all poisons, and such like.
>
> Said Dioscorides: Take walnuts before and after eating poison.
>
> It is reported of al-Mahdī that he said: I entered into the house of al-Manṣūr. I saw him eating walnuts & cheese. So, I said to him: What is this? And he said: My father told me of someone who once saw the Prophet eating cheese & walnuts. And he questioned him about it. And the Prophet replied: Cheese is a disease and walnuts are a medicine. If you combine the two, you have a remedy. This tradition is related in the al-Wasīla."[272]

Al-Dhahabī is thus clearly branching off from the earlier works of Prophetic Medicine in what pertains to his sources. He quite often mentions ʿAbd al-Laṭīf al-Baghdādī's *al-Arbaʿīn* as his source, but it was suggested by al-Nasīmī that he also used the *al-Aḥkām* of Ibn Ṭarkhān. Al-Nasīmī compared the phrasing from both works and concluded that they were too alike to be

---

[271] *Ibid.*, 73.
[272] *Ibid.*, 77-78.

unrelated.[273] Al-Dhahabī not only drew traditions from the six canonical compilations (the *Ṣaḥīḥs* of al-Bukhārī and Muslim, the *Sunans* of Abū Dā'ūd, Ibn Māja, al-Tirmidhī and al-Nisā'ī), but also from the *Sunan al-kubra* of al-Bayhaqī and the *Ṭibb al-nabī* of al-Iṣfahānī.[274] Finally, as we have seen with the last example, the author did not limit his sources to *ḥadīths*, but also included quotes from famous Greek physicians.

Of course, this extension of the material from which Prophetic Medicine was drawing also provoked a broadening of the medical content of the works. To take an example from al-Dhahabī, he lists medicaments that were never mentioned in earlier works of Prophetic Medicine, such as lavender (*usṭūkhūdus*)[275], anise (*anīsūn*)[276], and camomile (*bābūnaj*).[277]

This is also true for the third and final part of al-Dhahabī's work. In this part, the author presents specific diseases and their treatment as well as certain religious issues that pertain to medicine. Al-Dhahabī mentioned certain afflictions that were not presented in earlier texts but that were clearly common in his time, e.g. nosebleed (*ru'āf*), cough (*su'āl*) and colic (*qawlanj*).[278]

The third part of al-Dhahabī's work does not only present specific diseases, but also discusses different issues pertaining to medicine. Among these, he considers the matter of whether or not it is permissible to use medicine, as it was considered by certain ascetic believers that reliance on God ("*tawakkul*") was preferable. Indeed, to ascetics like Abū Dharr al-Ghifārī (d. 652)[279], a very early companion of the Prophet, illnesses were trials sent by God to test their fate,

---

273 Al-Nasīmī, *al-Ṭibb al-nabawī*, 1:83.
274 Perho, *The Prophet's Medicine*, 58.
275 *Ibid*., 69.
276 Elgood, *Tibb ul-Nabbi*, 70.
277 *Ibid*., 70-71.
278 Perho, *The Prophet's Medicine*, 58.
279 J.Robson, "Abū D̲h̲arr," in *Encyclopaedia of Islam*, 2nd edition, edited by P. Bearman, Th. Bianquis, C.E. Bosworth, E. van Donzel, W.P. Heinrichs, (Leiden: Brill, 2012), accessed May 11th, 2017, http://dx.doi.org/10.1163/1573-3912_islam_SIM_0173.

or graces bestowed by God upon the believer who received it as an opportunity to atone for his sins.[280] Furthermore, for the likes of Abū Dardā᾽ (d. 652), also a companion of the Prophet, it was considered useless to take medicaments and follow the recommendations of a physician because God only could ordain illness in a man, and only He could ordain health. This seems to have also been the opinion proffered by Abu Bakr al-Ṣiddīq (d. 634), first caliph of Islam.[281]

Authors of Prophetic Medicine objected to these opinions, based on many well-known traditions recorded in the *saḥiḥayn* (the *Saḥiḥ* of al-Bukhārī and that of Abū Muslim), that the Prophet enjoined Muslims to use medicaments as God had not given an illness for which he had not also given a cure, and it was common in the *sunna* of the Prophet to use medicaments.[282] Thus, the justification for the use of medicine was rooted in the accounts of the Prophet's use of medicine both local and foreign. Indeed, al-Dhahabī mentions a *ḥadīth* from ʿĀ᾽isha: "The Prophet had many illnesses. At such times there used to come and sit beside him several Arab and non-Arab doctors who gave him medicine."[283]

Al-Dhahabī also presents some of the traditions that support the principle of reliance on God, but gives his own opinion on the matter, siding with those that do not refuse medicine. He does, however, mention some reports according to which medicine is considered permissible, but abstinence from it is preferable on account of *ḥadīths* from al-Bukhārī and Abū Muslim stating that "A women came to the Prophet and said: O Prophet of God, ask God to cure me. And he said:

[280] Perho, *The Prophet's Medicine*, 65.
[281] *Ibid.*, 65-66.
[282] For example, see al-Bukhārī, *The Translation of the Meaning*, 395 (582).
[283] Elgood, *Tibb ul-Nabbi*, 124.

I will ask God if you wish it and He will cure you. But if you are willing to endure your sickness, you will gain Paradise. And the women said: O Prophet of God, nay rather, I will endure it."[284]

Al-Dhahabī not only supports his view that medicine should be permissible by revelation, but also through rational argument:

"The author of this book (upon whom may God show mercy) remarks that dependence means the reliance of the heart upon God. This is never contrary to reasons and causes and the majority of causes are subservient to dependence. So the skilful practitioner does what is proper and plans his reliance upon God in the final result."[285]

According to him, it is necessary that medical means be expended in order to bring about the recovery of an ill individual. However, the "final result", i.e. health, is only possible through the will of God. The realisation of the effects of medicine is subservient to whether or not God wills these effects to occur.

Another main issue taken up by al-Dhahabī is that of the study of medicine. As we have mentioned earlier and as has been suggested by Irmeli Perho, it is probable that one of the reasons behind the development of Prophetic Medicine is the lack of Muslim practitioners in the ranks of the physicians. Al-Dhahabī quotes al-Shāfiʿī:

> "After the Science which distinguishes between what is lawful and what is unlawful, I know of no Science which is more noble than Medicine. […] [Muslims] have lost one-third of human knowledge and have allowed themselves to be

---

[284] *Ibid.*, 125-126.
[285] *Ibid.*, 125.

replaced by Jews and Christians. [...] Verily the people of the Book have now conquered and surpassed us in this sublime Art."[286]

He follows this by *ḥadīths* that might encourage Muslims to take up the art of medicine, including many variations of the reports showing that ʿĀʾisha was well versed in medicine, that she learnt much of it from those that came to help the Prophet in his illnesses, and that the Prophet said that "He who gives medical care but is not recognised as a physician and thereby causes death or anything short of that, he is held responsible for this."[287]

On the issue of cauterisation, al-Dhahabī explains two contradicting positions based on verified *ḥadīths*. He cites many traditions that we have already mentioned from al-Bukhārī and others according to which the Prophet forbad cautery. He also cites reports attesting that the Prophet authorised the practice when the ailment "defeats the strongest of medicines and no drug succeeds."[288] Rather, al-Dhahabī advocates for a position in between: cauterisation is forbidden when it is seen as the *essential cause* of the recovery instead of the *occasion* of it, for indeed, only God can be the *essential cause*. It is instead acceptable, and even obligatory, in case of necessity, such as a prevention of haemorrhage which would be fatal or after the amputation of a hand or a foot.[289]

The matter of the Evil Eye is also taken up by al-Dhahabī. Al-Dhahabī's opinion supports not only the reality of the Eye, but also that of the effectiveness of reciting verses and wearing amulets against it. To justify this position, he cites *ḥadīths* reported by al-Bukhārī, Abū Muslim,

---

[286] *Ibid.*, 128-129.
[287] *Ibid.*, 130.
[288] *Ibid.*, 144-145.
[289] *Ibid.*, 146.

Ibn Māja, Abū Dāwūd, Mālik ibn Anas, and al-Tirmidhī.[290] While he cites many opinions concerning this matter, for al-Dhahabī incantations and charms are allowed and useful as they are "a form of taking refuge in God for the purpose of securing health."[291] However, these practices are considered blameworthy when they are not in Arabic and when the words are not understood. "The prohibition is directed against heretical charms,"[292] he explains, whereas calling upon God and His Prophet is not forbidden in itself.

Al-Dhahabī's approach to the matter of the incantations is interesting because it reveals a deeper theological engagement with medicine than his predecessors. While the first part of the book attempts to provide justification of Greek medical theory through Revelation, this third part of the work will often explain parts of the Revelation through Greek theory. For example, al-Dhahabī presents this *ḥadīth* from ʿĀʾisha:

> "When people used to complain of something such as an ulcer or a wound, the Prophet would put his finger to the dust. Then he would raise it and say: In the name of God, the dust of our earth united to the spittle of some of us will cure our sick with the permission of the Lord."[293]

Al-Dhahabī explains this quote thusly:

> "The phrase 'dust of our earth' is used because the constitution of dust is cold & dry and a desiccant for all damp. Now, ulcers and wounds contain much damp

[290] *Ibid.*, 152-154.
[291] *Ibid.*, 154.
[292] *Ibid.*
[293] *Ibid.*, 155.

within, which checks the good functioning of the Faculties and so hinders speedy healing."[294]

Here al-Dhahabī takes a well-known tradition from the Prophet and uses humoral theory to explain the words. This is significant as it strikingly demonstrates the extent of the assimilation of both medical traditions into each other.

Also of note is a brief section on spiritual cures. According to al-Dhahabī, and based on a *ḥadīth* from Abū Hurayra, prayer can be used to cure "pain in the heart, in the stomach and in the bowel."[295] There are three principles extracted from this. The first is the command to worship. The second is the psychological relief that prayer causes: when concentrated on the prayer, the believer overthrows the pain and casts it out. The third principle is that Prophetic Medicine is more holistic than its humoral counterpart: the doctor may prescribe prayer because it causes the patient to feel joy, grief, hope and fear, which in turn will "strengthen the faculties, delight the heart, and drive away disease by this very means."[296]

Praying is also presented as having physical benefits, for it contains many movements by which the joints of the body as well as the organs are moved and subsequently relaxed. This allows a hastening of the ejection of impurities.[297] The rest of the section on spiritual medicine lists different incantations that were used or recommended by the Prophet to cure certain ailments like insomnia, fever, chronic pain, etc. All the incantations evoke God and his prophets.[298]

---

294 *Ibid.*
295 *Ibid.*, 157.
296 *Ibid.*, 158.
297 *Ibid.*
298 *Ibid.*, 158-160.

The *al-Ṭibb al-nabawī* of Ibn Qayyim al-Jawziyya represents an even further phase of the encounter between Revelation and medicine. As we will see, it is very similar in form to the work of his contemporary al-Dhahabī, but it presents an even further adaptation of the Graeco-Islamic medical theory in order to make it comply with more specific tenets of religion.

Determining the objectives of a text is often an arduous task, and one that must be undertaken with sensitivity. However, it may be possible to grasp some of it by looking closely at the context, which we have attempted in the previous chapter, and confronting it to the content. The intended public of a work of Prophetic Medicine like that of Ibn Qayyim al-Jawziyya was wide-ranging, and included both specialized scholars and physicians, but especially the general public. After all, the *al-Ṭibb al-nabawī* of Ibn Qayyim al-Jawziyya consisted of the medical chapters of his *Zād al-maʿād fī hadī khayr al-ʿibād Muḥammad* ("Provisions for the Hereafter on the Guidance of the Best of Servants, Muhammad"), a work dedicated to publicizing the author's opinion of correct behaviour, and described by Perho as an "exhortative *bidʿa* ("innovation") tract".[299] It included practical advice on many aspects of Muslims' daily life, including rituals, legal topics, social conduct, etc.[300] It aimed at warning the public about what should be considered impious and exhorted the readers to respect what he considered correct behaviour. To him, for a Muslim, being informed on the life of the Prophet allows for a better emulation, and enables virtue, which in turn enables salvation.

[299] Perho, *The Prophet's Medicine*, 30.
[300] Irmeli Perho, "Ibn Qayyim al-Ǧawziyyah's Contribution to the Prophet's Medicine," *Oriente Moderno* 90 (2010), 191.

In his *al-Ṭibb al-nabawī*, Ibn Qayyim al-Jawziyya's stated intention was to disseminate the guidance of the Prophet concerning medical issues so that Muslims may do what God enjoins, and avoid what He forbids:

> "We shall merely give an indication of all of this, for the Messenger of God (p.b.u.h) was sent as a guide to call people to God and His Paradise, and to give knowledge of God, making clear to the Community what pleases Him and commanding them accordingly, and what angers Him and forbidding them accordingly; to teach them about the prophets and messengers, and their lives within their respective communities, and about the creation of the world, about the beginning and the end, and that which causes suffering or happiness for mankind."[301]

It is divided into two parts. The first part consists of two chapters in which we find a presentation of medical theory highly indebted to the works of Galen and physicians of the Hippocratic legacy, and that quite resembles the first part of the work of al-Dhahabī.

However, Ibn Qayyim al-Jawziyya clearly gives precedence to the guidance of the Prophet over that of the physicians concerning medicine. Indeed, in his introduction, he states that the wisdom of the medical sayings of the Prophet "is not accessible to the intellects of the greatest of physicians."[302] He thus uses the Qur'ān as a basis to categorize diseases: first there are the sicknesses of the heart (*qalb*), then the sicknesses of the body. The principle of sickness of the heart is based on the many passages of the Qur'ān: "The Most High has said: 'In their hearts is a

---

[301] Ibn Qayyim al-Jawziyya, *Medicine of the Prophet*, 17.
[302] *Ibid.*, 3.

disease; and Allāh has increased their disease' (II:10)"[303] There are two kinds of sicknesses of the heart: uncertainty and doubt (*shubha wa-shakk*), and desire and temptation (*shahwa wa-ghayy*).[304] Obtaining knowledge pertaining to medicine of the heart is not possible without the Messengers of God. This type of medicine is thus not the affair of physicians, because "the tranquility of the heart is obtained through recognition of its Lord and Creator, His Names and Attributes, His actions and judgements; and it should prefer what He approves of and loves, and should avoid what He forbids and dislikes."[305]

It must be acknowledged that despite these cases that we have mentioned, more often than not, the Galenic medical theory mostly did not contradict the Prophet's word. Ibn Qayyim al-Jawziyya's conceptualization of the relation between the Prophet's medicine and that of the physicians is that the first is superior to the latter:

> "We would say that the connection between the medicine of the Messengers and that of the physicians is as tenuous as [the physicians' medicine's] connection with the medicine of village healers."[306]

However, to him, while the sacredness of revealed knowledge was unequivocal, the medicine of the physicians, obtained through empiricism, experiment and deduction, was not unacceptable. Ibn Qayyim al-Jawziyya often refers to Galen as the "most excellent physician" and quotes his works and that of Hippocrates[307] and Arab physicians like al-Rāzī on various subjects.[308] He also refers to Jibrīl ibn Bukhtīshūʿ (d. 827), physician to Hārūn al-Rashīd (d. 809) and al-

303 *Ibid.*, 3-4.
304 *Ibid.*
305 *Ibid.*, 5.
306 *Ibid.*, 8.
307 For example, concerning the effect of seasons on health, he quotes Hippocrates' *Airs, Waters, Places*. *Ibid.*, 30.
308 For example, concerning the treatment of fever with cold water, he quotes al-Rāzī's *al-Ḥāwī fī al-ṭibb*, *Ibid.*, 19.

Ma'mūn (d. 833), concerning the harmfulness of the combination of eggs and fish,[309] and Yūḥannā ibn Māsawayh (d. 857), who worked as director of the hospital of Baghdad and was physician to al-Ma'mūn, concerning the citron (*utrujj*).[310] On indigofera (*katam*), he quotes the philosopher Ya'qūb ibn Isḥāq al-Kindī (d. 873), author of a formulary of compound medicines;[311] on food and drink he quotes Thābit ibn Qurra (d. 901);[312] on forbidden substances, he quotes 'Alī ibn al-'Abbās al-Majūsī (d. 944), author of *Kāmil al-ṣinā'a al-ṭibbiyya* ("Perfection in the Art of Medicine");[313] on the constellation of the Pleiades, he quotes Abū 'Abd-Allāh Muḥammad ibn Aḥmad ibn Sa'īd al-Tamīmī (d. 980);[314] on camel's milk, he quotes Isḥāq ibn Sulaymān al-Isrā'īlī (d. 950), who worked as a physician, oculist and philosopher in Cairo and Tunisia;[315] on ophtalmia (*ramad*), he quotes the physician and oculist Sharaf al-Dīn 'Alī ibn 'Īsā al-Kaḥḥal (d. after 1010);[316] on the use of clay for ulcers, Ibn Qayyim al-Jawziyya quotes Abū Sahl 'Īsā ibn Yaḥyỳ al-Masīḥī al-Jurjānī (d. 1010);[317] on the use of the fruit of salvadora persica (*kabāth*), he quotes Abū al-Ḥasan 'Alī ibn Riḍwān (d. 1068), physician to al-Mustanṣir (d. 1094) in Egypt.[318] He quotes from Andalusian physician Ibn Zuhr (Avenzoar) (d. 1162) on the toothbrush (*siwāk*) and narcissus (*narjis*).[319] Ibn Qayyim al-Jawziyya also quotes from three Andalusian botanists: Sulaymān ibn al-Ḥasan ibn Juljul (d. after 994) on salvadora persica,[320] Ibn Samajūn, contemporary to Ibn Juljul on aloes

[309] *Ibid*., 283.
[310] *Ibid*., 205.
[311] *Ibid*., 259.
[312] *Ibid*., 151.
[313] *Ibid*., 119.
[314] *Ibid*., 30.
[315] *Ibid*., 34.
[316] *Ibid*., 81.
[317] *Ibid*., 140.
[318] *Ibid*., 259.
[319] *Ibid*., 231, 279.
[320] *Ibid*.

wood (*ʿūd*),[321] and Abū Jaʿfar Aḥmad ibn Muḥammad al-Ghāfiqī (d. 1135), author of a large herbal, on citron, truffles (*kamaʿa*), and indigofera.[322]

The medicine of the physicians was, however, incomplete, mostly because it did not encompass the health of the heart and the soul, and because it was not based on divine guidance:

> "If anyone does not distinguish between the one and the other [medicine of the heart and medicine of the body], he should weep over the life of his heart, as it should be counted among the dead, and over its light, for it is submerged in the seas of darkness."[323]

Furthermore, Ibn Qayyim al-Jawziyya states that spiritual health, as well as health of the heart, is more important, and health of the body is contingent upon it. "Restoration of the body without restoration of the heart is of no benefit," he explains, "whereas damage to the body while the spirit is restored brings limited harm, for it is a temporary damage which will be followed by a permanent and complete cure."[324]

To him, the medicine of the body is of two types: that which may be treated by their simple opposites, and that which require thought. The first type includes the treatment of hunger and thirst, cold, weariness, etc. The cause of a bodily illness is a departure from the balance of the temperaments (*mizāj*). This is itself either material, i.e. from an internal cause (*māddiyya*), qualitative, i.e. upsetting the constitution (*kayfiyya*) and producing a condition, or organic, i.e. in a limb or organ (*āliyya*).[325] A material illness is when there occurs an excessive increase in a

---

[321] *Ibid.*, 244.
[322] *Ibid.*, 205, 259-260.
[323] *Ibid.*, 5.
[324] *Ibid.*, 17.
[325] *Ibid.*, 6.

substance in the body, and is most often caused by "consuming more food before the previous meal has been properly digested; by eating in excess of the amount needed by the body; by taking in food which is of little nutritional value and slow to digest; and by indulging in different foods which are complex in their composition."[326] A qualitative illness is when "the matter that actually caused it have ceased to exist, for while these matters abate, their effect remains as a condition within the temperament."[327]

Ibn Qayyim al-Jawziyya did not describe the main principle of medicine of the body in the same way that contemporary medical books did. To him, the principles were "preservation of health, protection from harm and expulsion of corrupt substances."[328] In a contemporary medical textbook, the principles were the "preservation of health, and its restoration when disturbed."[329] The addition of the "expulsion of corrupt substances" as one of the main principles of bodily medicine stems from a verse of the Qur'ān (II:196) which allows the believers to make ritual compensation if they have an ailment in their head. His interpretation is that this was to allow them to shave their heads to "evacuate the harmful vapours that brought the ailment on his head through being congested beneath the hair."[330] Ibn Qayyim al-Jawziyya uses analogy to expand this passage to ten things that cause harm if retained or repressed: "blood when it is agitated, semen when it is moving, urine, feces, wind, vomiting, sneezing, sleep, hunger, thirst."[331] To explain this usage of the meaning of the verse, the author explains that "such is the method of the Qur'ān: to give instruction about the greater, through mentioning the lesser."[332]

---

326 *Ibid.*, 12-13.
327 *Ibid.*, 6.
328 *Ibid.*, 4.
329 *Ibid.*
330 *Ibid.*, 4.
331 *Ibid.*, 5.
332 *Ibid.*

In an admittedly short passage, Ibn Qayyim al-Jawziyya tackled the issue of the relation of the medicine of the physicians to the Revelation. Prophetic Medicine heals "certain illnesses that even the minds of the great physicians cannot grasp, and which their science, experiments and analogical deductions cannot reach."[333] Obviously, the author did not refute the entirety of the medicine of the physicians. However, he did refute the assertion that it was all-encompassing and that it could be an absolute system: the medicine of the physicians, along with its main methods, i.e. experiments, deductions, and analogy, cannot be complete without the medical prescriptions of God and His Messenger. Here, Ibn Qayyim al-Jawziyya does not refute the use of reason in medicine. Rather, he points out that the completeness of a system of medicine is contingent on both types of sources of medical knowledge: experiment and deduction on the one hand, which is associated with Greek-inherited medical theory, and religion on the other, which is represented by the Revelation.

In the same way, Ibn Qayyim al-Jawziyya does not take at face value the Greek explanation of the components of the body. Contrary to al-Dhahabī and the medical theory that he followed in his work, he states that the human body is made up of earth, air, and water, and it is for this reason that the Prophet had talked about food, drink, and breath:

> "In the *Musnad* and elsewhere it is reported that the Prophet (p.b.u.h) said: 'The human being can fill no container worse than his belly. Sufficient for the son of Adam are so many morsels as will keep his spine upright. But if he must eat more, then a third for his food, a third for his drink and a third for his breath.'"[334]

---

[333] *Ibid.*, 8.
[334] *Ibid.*, 12-13.

Thus, Ibn Qayyīm al-Jawziyya does not accept the physicians' claim that there is a part of fire in the human body. To justify his position, he gives four arguments to prove not only that there is not a fiery component in the human body, but also not in plants and animals. Firstly, to the claim that the fiery component descended from the upper spheres[335], he answers that fire by nature rises, so it could not have descended, especially because it would have needed to pass through the sphere of intense coldness (*zamharīr*).[336]

Secondly, to the claim that the fiery component was created amongst the watery, airy and earthy components of the body, he answers that fire could not have appeared in a body because it would have been transformed or extinguished by its greater quantity of watery components.[337]

Thridly, the Quʾran contains specific information about the creation of man by God. In some places, God says that man was created from water (XXXII:8), earth (III:59, XVIII:37), or clay, i.e. a mixture of water and earth (VII:12). The Qurʾān never mentions that God created man from fire. Iblīs, i.e. Satan, however, is said to have been created from fire (XXXVIII:76, LV:15).[338]

Finally, to Ibn Qayyim al-Jawziyya, that there exists heat in the body of humans and animals is not an indication of there being fire, "for heat can be caused by things other than fire. Sometimes it comes from fire, at other times from motion, and from the reflection of rays, from heat of the air and from the proximity of fire [...] through the medium of the air."[339] The rejection of fire as an element did not warrant a rejection of the whole medical system based on the humors. "On a theoretical level," explains Perho, "there was a connection between the elements and the

---

[335] The Greek cosmological model of the celestial spheres realizes the universe as a set of geocentric spheres. Earth is in the sublunary sphere, beyond which is the *aether*, where the planets are located.
[336] Ibn Qayyim al-Jawziyya, *Medicine of the Prophet*, 13-14.
[337] *Ibid.*, 15.
[338] *Ibid.*
[339] *Ibid.*

humors, but it was the humors that were important in determining aetiology, defining illnesses and choosing therapies."[340]

The rest of the first part of the treatise is composed of 36 other chapters mainly describing treatments for specific ailments such as fever, diarrhea, plague, dropsy, wounds, pleurisy, headache, cardiac pain, ophthalmia, lice, the Evil Eye, etc. It also presents specific treatments, their justification and their use, such as cupping, fasting, incantations, etc.[341] The great majority of justification, proofs, and details concerning the treatments mentioned here are based on religious reasons, and refer to the Qur'ān and to the *sunna*.

Ibn Qayyim al-Jawziyya sometimes uses the discussion of a certain illness to demonstrate the superiority of the revelation, as is the case with plague and the effects of evil spirits and the like. He accepts that the "corruption of the air" is among the causes of plague, as explained by the physicians, but he stresses that they cannot give information about hidden matters and spiritual beings.[342]

As for the second part of the work, it consists of an extensive alphabetical list of simple foods and drugs. Authors of Prophetic Medicine do not include compounds in their lists and mention that diet is preferable over medicaments, and that simples are preferable over compounds, but they do not reject their use. Ibn Qayyim al-Jawziyya mentions that simples are sometimes completed with that which will reinforce or temper their strength, but does not discuss this further.[343] He also explains, as Ibn Khaldūn did in his *Muqaddima*, that "city-dwellers, whose food

340 Perho, "Ibn Qayyim al-Ǧawziyyah's Contribution", 202.
341 Ibn Qayyim al-Jawziyya, *Medicine of the Prophet*, 17-204.
342 *Ibid.*, 28-29.
343 *Ibid.*, 7.

is mostly composite, need compound medicines,"[344] while "Bedouin and desert dwellers suffer from simple illnesses, so for their medication simple drugs suffice."[345]

Concerning compounds, al-Dhahabī is of the same opinion, but he does present some examples of compounds, the components of which often serve the purpose of changing the taste of a simple that would be unpleasant, or that of slowing or accelerating its effect, or that of increasing or decreasing its potency, depending on the characteristic of the illness.[346]

Ibn Qayyim al-Jawziyya's list of drugs and foodstuffs presents substances and practices in the same way as al-Dhahabī; along with extensive quotations of *ḥadīths* that support or mention the usage of the substances, their humoral essential qualities (hot, cold, dry, moist) are presented. This thusly forms a system of medicine that is both allopathic, i.e. treating a condition with its opposite, and revelational. However, while al-Dhahabī's work included substances for which there was no support from *ḥadīth*, Ibn Qayyim al-Jawziyya's list is more reliant on revealed medicine than it is on the humoral qualities of the substances.

The differences we have mentioned between the work of al-Dhahabī and that of Ibn Qayyim al-Jawziyya are telling. Al-Dhahabī's work took up the legacy of al-Baghdādī and Ibn Ṭarkhān and systematized the medical utterances of the Prophet. *Al-Ṭibb al-nabawī* of Ibn Qayyim al-Jawziyya not only merged further the two traditions, i.e. the medicine of the physicians and that of the Prophet, but actively engaged with the theory that earlier authors of Prophetic medicine had not questioned. In his explanation of the main principles of medicine, his discussion of the relationship between the Prophet's medical knowledge and that of the physicians, his arguments

---

[344] *Ibid.*, 8.
[345] *Ibid.*; Ibn Khaldūn, *The Muqaddimah: an Introduction to History*, trans. Franz Rosenthal, ed. N. J. Dawood (Princeton and Oxford: Princeton University Press, 1967), 387.
[346] Elgood, *Tibb ul-Nabbī*, 119-120.

concerning the elements, his more extensive use of *ḥadīths* to discuss specific drugs and foodstuff, Ibn Qayyim al-Jawziyya breaks from the tradition of Prophetic Medicine. In his Prophetic Medicine, he points to doctrinally controversial issues of medical theory that he thought needed modifications in order to be theologically acceptable to the Muslim community.

Later works of Prophetic Medicine tended to stick more closely to the earlier texts of the genre. Ibn Qayyim al-Jawziyya's disciple, the Ḥanbalī Jamāl al-Dīn al-Surramarrī (d. 1374) authored a treatise of Prophetic Medicine entitled *Kitāb shifā' al-ālām fī ṭibb ahl al-islam* ("The Book on Curing of Pains in the Medicine of the People of Islam"), which was predominantly a handbook on common foodstuffs.[347] He divided his work in the same way that al-Dhahabī had done: a part on theory, one on medicaments and foodstuffs, and a last one on symptoms and cures.

Two physicians from Yemen need to be mentioned as they were authors of books on the medicine of the Prophet: Mahdī ibn ʿAlī ibn Ibrāhīm al-Ṣanawbarī al-Yamanī (d. 1412) and Ibrāhīm ibn ʿAbd al-Raḥmān ibn Abī Bakr al-Azraq (d. 1485). Al-Ṣanawbarī's work, *Kitāb al-raḥma fī al-ṭibb wa-al-ḥikma* ("The Book of Mercy in Medicine and Wisdom"), and that of al-Azraq, *Kitāb tashīl al-manāfiʿ fī al-ṭibb wa-al-ḥikam* ("The Book on the Benefits of Medicine and Wisdom Made Accessible"), only succinctly discussed medical theory, and focused on practical advices based on both the Prophet's guidance and the works of Hippocrates, Galen and al-Rāzī.[348]

The already mentioned treatise of Ibn Mufliḥ, *al-Ādāb al-sharʿiyya wa-al-minaḥ al-marʿiyya*, followed the theoretical and theological views of Ibn Qayyim al-Jawziyya without citing him directly, but he did avoid certain discussions of medical theory that did not correspond to

[347] Perho, "Ibn Qayyim al-Ǧawziyyah's Contribution," 209.
[348] Perho, *The Prophet's Medicine*, 59-60.

Islamic doctrine. For example, he did not question the theory of the four elements and the presence of fire in the human body; he instead directly discussed the resulting temperaments.[349]

The work of Jalāl al-Dīn al-Suyūṭī (d. 1505) titled a*l-Manhaj al-sawī wa-al-manhal al-rawī fī al-ṭibb al-nabawī*[350] ("The Correct Method and the Thirst-quenching Spring of the Prophet's Medicine"), relates more to the earlier compilation of medical *ḥadīths* than it does to the works of al-Dhahabī and Ibn Qayyim al-Jawziyya. The medical content of the sayings is not discussed, and the focus is put on regrouping a large number of traditions.[351]

Another later work, the *al-Manhal al-rawī fī al-ṭibb al-nabawī* ("The Thirst-quenching Spring of the Prophet's Medicine") of Shams al-Dīn Muḥammad ibn ʿAlī Ibn Ṭūlūn al-Dimashqī (d. 1546) quoted Ibn Qayyim al-Jawziyya but did not mention his discussions of medical theories, and provided only limited comments and explanation of the *ḥadīths* he presented. Thus, "the result of Ibn Ṭūlūn's method", explains Perho, "is that both revealed and rational knowledge remain segregated and no coherent synthesis emerges."[352]

The evolution of Prophetic Medicine that we outlined here allows us to grasp some details of the way Greek medical theory was combined with the Prophet's utterances concerning medicine. From the early years of Islam to the 15th century, what came to be known as Prophetic Medicine emerged as simple uncommented topical collections of sayings and developed into its own genre of medico-religious literature.

---

349 Perho, "Ibn Qayyim al-Ǧawziyyah's Contribution," 201-202.
350 Jalāl al-Dīn al-Suyūṭī, *al-Manhaj al-sawī wa-al-manhal al-rawī fī al-ṭibb al-nabawī*, (Beirut: Mu'assasat al-Kutūb al-Thaqāfiyya, 1986).
351 Perho, *The Prophet's Medicine,* 61.
352 Perho, "Ibn Qayyim al-Ǧawziyyah's Contribution," 210.

From an assortment of seemingly disordered Prophetic reports, it was expanded and transformed into a stand-alone medical system that did not quite intend to replace the medicine of the contemporary physicians, but that also could not allow it, for theological reasons, to continue as it was. This was not a complete overhaul of the principles of medicine as it was known and practiced and as it continued to be, but it demonstrated that some scholars of the *ahl al-ḥadīth* saw the importance of engaging with this tradition and reiterating the precedence of Islamic doctrine in all spheres of Muslim life.

The significance of *al-Ṭibb al-nabawī* of Ibn Qayyim al-Jawziyya is that it represented the ultimate merging of Greek medical theory and Prophetic medical sayings into a compromised medical system. This medical system, as indebted to Galenic medical theory as it was, stressed the importance of the Revelation and attempted to adjust theoretical issues so that it becomes theologically acceptable for all Muslims. Ibn Qayyim al-Jawziyya attempted to coherently join the two traditions in order to create something that would not, contrary to the currently accepted medical theory of his contemporaries, go against the prescriptions of God and Messenger.

By the 14th century, the genre of Prophetic Medicine had thus evolved from mere compilations of the Prophet's words and actions that had to do with medicine and health, to a critical engagement of the piety of Muslims with a centuries-old tradition of medicine.

CONCLUSION

The aim of this thesis has been to fill a gap that the modern historiography of Prophetic Medicine had left, particularly on the subject of the nature of this genre of religious medical literature. The gap, as we identified it, stems from a certain way of studying science in Islam that focused on the Greek heritage present in treatises of Prophetic Medicine. The early scholarship on the subject, like that of Manfred Ullmann and Christoph Bürgel, had pictured Prophetic Medicine as an attempt by religious scholars to react and provide an alternative to the medicine of foreign origin. This alternative was aimed to replace Greek-based medicine by a set of practices sanctified by the *ḥadīths* and consequently doctrinally imperative. The studies of Michael Dols and Irmeli Perho had presented a more positive view of Prophetic Medicine. To them, Prophetic Medicine was an Islamic appropriation of the content of Greek medical heritage. In the light of what we have shown in this thesis, it appears evident that these later authors were very close to the mark in their definition of Prophetic Medicine, and their characterization of the intentions of the authors was the most comprehensive assessment yet. However, in both cases, with the early studies as well as with the reaction of later authors, the method of investigating the intentions of Prophetic Medicine had lacked contextualization. As revisionist historiography had accomplished in the 80s and 90s with Islamic science in general, it had proven that the authors of Prophetic Medicine in particular had not rejected the principles of the Ancient sciences. A great accomplishment indeed, but it presented limitations in that it fixated on what Prophetic Medicine owed to the Greek physicians like Hippocrates and Galen. The old "Orientalist" literature, simply put, had the Enlightenment-old problem of seeing only the opposition of revelation and reason, but the extensive studies of

Prophetic Medicine, like that of Irmeli Perho, had focused too much on proving the acceptance of Greek "rational" medicine by authors of the genre.

When we take a step back from this long-standing clash between the reason vs revelation scheme on the one hand, and the revisionist framework on the other, we allow ourselves to go beyond the question of the Greek heritage of Prophetic Medicine. What is left for us is to look at the actual context of the centuries that saw the rise of Prophetic Medicine, as well as its origin throughout the history of Islam, and how this affected the content.

In the first chapter, we have shown that Galenic medicine was far from atheistic, and comprised many characteristics that made it possible to be adopted and adapted in a medical system related to a monotheistic faith, and we have made some observation concerning the readiness of Islam to receive Greek medicine and make it its own.

In the second chapter, we have looked at how the political, religious and intellectual background of the 11th to the 14th centuries had made it possible for a medicine based on the actions and the sayings of the Prophet to develop and thrive. The period was marked by some major political setbacks, like the Crusades, the Spanish Reconquista, and the Mongol invasions. However, intellectual activity was vibrant in cities like Damascus and Cairo, as part of a movement of institutionalization of scholarship and the development of establishment of learning. The new ruling elite's policies and way of life supported the growth of the intellectual class, but provoked certain critiques from religious scholars of the "traditionalist" camp; it also fostered a sentiment favorable to a "*Sunnī* revival" and a return to a stricter version of Islam.

The third chapter put the evolution of Prophetic Medicine under the looking glass, and approached it through a theoretical model of four stages. The first stage, taking place between the

8th and the 9th centuries, is represented by the "proto-Prophetic Medicine" found in the *ḥadīths* collections of the *Saḥīḥ* movement, which tried to guarantee the authenticity of the reports of the Prophet and arranged them according to their theme. Thus, the Prophetic Medicine of this era was embodied in chapters of collections like the *Kitāb al-Marḍā* ("The Book of the Sick") and the *Kitāb al-Ṭibb* ("The Book of Medicine") of the *Saḥīḥ al-Bukhārī*. The second stage, between the 10th and the 12th centuries, represents the moment where compilations of medical *ḥadīths* shifted their internal organization to match that of medical books of the period. This is significant because it suggests a change in the intentions and the target audience of Prophetic Medicine. Prophetic Medicine was henceforth not only the concern of *ḥadīth* scholars and jurists, but also that of physicians. The third stage, taking place between the 12th and the 13th centuries, saw the rise of treatises that combined the reports of the Prophet concerning medicine to the medical theory of "academic" and Greek-inspired medicine. Prophetic Medicine had thus properly become a genre of medical literature, as opposed to one of religious literature interested in medicine. The fourth stage, between the 13th and the 14th centuries, is the stage during which Prophetic Medicine matures and is most prolific. It is also the stage during which a relatively comprehensive medical system is established based both on Galen's principles and on the Islamic revelation. Certain authors of this era even confronted some of the contradictions that such a dual system of medicine exacerbated, as was the case of Ibn Qayyim al-Jawziyya and his discussion of the element of fire.

The way Prophetic Medicine has evolved and the context that surrounded its evolution makes apparent two observations: the first observation is that the authors generally did not reject the content of Greek medicine and did not hesitate to quote the names of the Greek physicians. The second observation, however, is that Prophetic Medicine did indeed mature into a critical engagement of religious traditionist scholars and Muslim physicians with the heritage of the

Greeks. Thus, instead of a question of whether this genre accepted or rejected the medicine of Galen, one must understand that the authors of Prophetic Medicine were open to it and found a way to adapt it to their faith, and to present a critical version of it that was adequate for the everyday life of the believers. We must not see Prophetic Medicine as a genre of religious literature that objected to the medical practice of their contemporaries, but rather as a genre of medical literature that objected to the uncritical "academic" medical literature that did not pause to question itself.

These considerations raise certain questions that could be pursued in the future, namely the reaction of the doctors of the "proper" Greco-Islamic medical tradition to the development of Prophetic Medicine, and their answers to such critiques as those of Ibn Qayyim al-Jawziyya concerning, for example, the presence of the element of fire in the body.

As stated above, *al-Ṭibb al-nabawī* of Ibn Qayyim al-Jawziyya was a later publishing of the medical chapters of his *Zād al-maʿād fī hadī khair al-ʿibād Muḥammad*, a work that advocated correct behavior and warned against impiety. We have mentioned earlier some elements of the moral aspect of Prophetic Medicine, but this could represent a scholarly endeavor of its own. However, it is with this context in mind that we have advocated for a modification of the opinions of Rahman, Dols and Perho. Prophetic Medicine presents indeed characteristics that proves that it did not aim at competing with contemporary medical practice that was based on the Greek heritage, but it is also part of an earlier tradition of *ḥadīths* compilation and a context of reaffirmation of traditionalism.

What this thesis has shown is the necessity of a critical look at the revisionist historiography of Prophetic Medicine. We have hereby presented an account of it that stresses the importance of contextualization in religious (the development of *ḥadīth* literature) and historical (the rise of the

Seljūks and Mamlūks) contexts. Keeping in mind the relation between the content of these works and the Greek medical heritage, we must also consider that Prophetic Medicine might have been something in between the portrayal of Bürgel and Ullmann on the one hand, and that of Rahman, Dols, and Perho on the other hand. It is not a matter of compete or complete, but something in between. The study of content has polarized modern authors into seeing "Hellenistic" medicine and Islamic doctrine as two elements in a clash, but contextualization helps us adopt a middle ground position and understand that Prophetic Medicine was the result of a very long evolution, and that it represented the more complex interactions of religion and science.

Milton Keynes UK
Ingram Content Group UK Ltd.
UKHW020926201123
432908UK00021B/3174

9 787458 208998